CW01647493

Emergency Wellbeing

written by a Firefighter

EMERGENCY WELLBEING

Contents

Part Four: Emotions Fading Fast

Part Five: Taking Back Control

Part Six: Small Steps

© 2022 Paul Casey

All rights reserved. No part of this book may be reproduced by any mechanical, photographic or electronic process, or in the form of a phonographic recording: nor may it be stored in a retrieval system, be transmitted or copied for public or private use, other than for 'fair use' as brief quotations embodied in articles and reviews, without prior written permission of the publisher.

The information given in this book should not be treated as a substitute for professional medical advice; always consult a medical practitioner. Any use of information within this book is at the reader's discretion and risk. Neither the publisher nor I can be held responsible for any loss, claim or damage arising out of the use, or misuse, of the suggestions made, the failure to take medical advice or for any material on third-party websites.

Some names and identifying details have been changed to protect the privacy of the individuals mentioned in this book. Although the author and publisher have made every effort to ensure that the information in this book was correct at time of press, the author and publisher do not assume and hereby disclaim any liability to any party for any loss, damage, or disruption caused by errors or omissions, whether such errors or omissions result from negligence, accident, or any other cause.

@EmergWellbeing

emergency_wellbeing

Please follow Emergency Wellbeing on social media for inspirational updates and to share your own stories of healing.

ISBN: 978-1-3999-2382-8

Introduction

'Everyone you meet is fighting a battle you know nothing about. Be kind. Always'

Robin Williams

If you've given your very precious time to start reading this book then, like me, you care about welfare. More importantly, your welfare. At the time of writing this book, I am a firefighter serving in the UK fire and rescue service. I am in the role of a Station Commander, a middle manager in charge of staff and assets within the service. I joined in 2005 and have worked across a number of different roles and ranks prior to my current position. For years I neglected my mental health and wellbeing. Only now do I take the time, make the effort and give wellbeing the attention it truly deserves.

Many roles within the emergency services are extremely stressful. Unfortunately, trauma, suffering, ill health and death, all form part of that normality. Albeit, not written exclusively for people who work within this sector; this book will give you an insight into the world of the fire and rescue service. A sample of what the knock-on effect can be from the constant exposure to stressful situations.

I feel I have an opportunity to share my story and help people who may be suffering in silence. I hope reading this book helps you find your pathway to a calmer sense of wellbeing, as it has me and that it provides you with a clearer understanding of how mental health issues can affect all of us differently.

Part One: What Have I Signed Up For?

Heart Racing

I had just drifted off to sleep. I had probably been asleep for around half an hour or so. I woke up to a very familiar sound, my fire service pager had activated. This loud tone was informing me that I needed to respond quickly to an emergency call.

I worked at a full-time fire station where the firefighter's houses backed onto the boundary of the fire station. I had five minutes in which to wake up, get out of bed, gather my senses, run over to the station, put on my fire kit and get on the fire engine (known as a pump) alongside three of my colleagues. My heart was racing, pounding out of my chest, as it often did when I was woken up suddenly in the middle of the night.

It was a very cold night with a mist hanging in the air. Once on the pump and ready to go, the officer in charge, who sat in the front, told us we were responding to an RTA. RTA 'Road Traffic Accident'. The terminology has since changed to RTC, 'Road Traffic Collison' because in the world of insurance and blame the term 'accident' means no one can be held accountable.

The RTC was reported to involve multiple vehicles and a double decker coach. The crash was on a slip road of the M4 motorway, right near Junction 16 of the M25. Reports coming in over the radio indicated that multiple people were trapped, and fatalities were believed to be involved.

I will pause the story for just a minute, to briefly tell you a little bit more about myself at that time. The year was 2007, it was the 4th of January and I had been a serving firefighter for exactly two years to the day. Just out of my probation period and now classed as 'competent', having completed all my practical training assessments and an NVQ (National Vocational Qualification) in Fire Service Operations as part of my training and development. Alongside me on the pump that night, was a driver, an officer in charge and another firefighter, like me, who had also just completed his probation. The driver and officer in charge, also competent firefighters had both already completed a number of years in service and were classed as old hands. I was 25 years old at the time of this particular incident and had been attending a number of other operational 'jobs' throughout my two years in the service.

The blue light drive to the incident was quiet with none of us really talking. We could hear over the radio reports that the ambulance service were already on scene and that this was being treated as a major incident. This ramped things up for us, we now knew that it was likely to be a big job. We would be arriving very soon, probably within the next five minutes, and we would potentially be the first pump on scene. This puts a lot of pressure on the first crew to arrive, to risk assess and instigate a plan to ensure the rescue of as many people as possible. We call this a casualty centred rescue, where our prime focus is on saving as many saveable lives as possible with the equipment and training we have. Unfortunately, on occasions when the fire service arrives first, where many multiple casualties may be involved, this can mean sometimes mean we are put in the position of having to play 'god' and prioritise our efforts on who we believe can be saved.

Every firefighter is given basic first aid training, and for most this is enhanced to a level similar to an ambulance technician, which means we have the training to be able to triage casualties and determine who needs to be helped first, dependant on injury severity. When the casualty numbers outweigh the number of firefighters on scene this can prove to be overwhelming even for the most experienced crews.

Thoughts of what I might see on arrival raced through my mind on our final approach to the scene. How many people will be suffering? How challenging a rescue effort will this be for me? Then we were there.

The motorway slip road was eerily quiet. I could see a few lights in the distance, the blue lights of two ambulances and another pump that had already arrived on scene. I remember thinking 'phew, thank god we were not first' and that we had some help with what we might be faced with. I got off the pump and remember the cold air of the night filling my lungs and the potent smell of oil and diesel fumes engulfing me.

What I saw ahead of me, once my eyes focused and the dim orange glow of the halogen motorway streetlights lit the road, I will never forget. This image is ingrained into my mind, even now years later, and I'm sure it will stay with me throughout my life on this planet. I saw a large double decker coach, I could only make out the roof, as it was laying on its side. I could hear faint screams from people trapped inside, people were wandering in the road, zombie like, dazed and confused not sure where to go or what to do. Some looked ok to me, others, such as those laying on the slip road covered in blood looked worse. I felt I was stood on the same spot forever taking in and absorbing the horror that was before me. In reality it was probably only for a few seconds. Standing there and looking around those seconds felt like they had slowed down into hours. A cliché I know, but a genuine and bizarre loss of my grip on time and reality for a few seconds.

The officer in charge of my pump had ran up to the coach and was liaising with the other emergency services already in attendance and putting together a plan. A middle-aged man had started to walk towards me, holding his head, his shirt was covered in blood. He stared at me, his eyes locked on mine as he inched closer, I could see he had taken a very severe head injury and had been scalped along the side of his face up to the top of his head. I had to help him, and my training took over, I told him to lay down in front of me, I shouted to my colleague to bring the first aid pack over to me. I asked the man for his name and what happened, he mumbled something in response that I couldn't make out. I knew he was in pain, but apart from a mumbled reply he was very quiet. I knew this could be a bad sign. Casualties becoming unresponsive can mean their injury is worse than it physically appears.

I remember watching an old army recruitment advert on television which stuck in my head. Which casualty you should treat first? It asked. The one screaming, or the silent one. It was the latter.

My colleague dropped the first aid bag at my feet, I applied a bandage to the man's head to try and stem the bleeding. I wanted to put him on oxygen to help calm him and increase his oxygen levels which are often low after losing blood.

Suddenly I could hear someone shouting at me, it was a paramedic, he was with a woman who looked to be in complete shock.

He shouted again "She can't find her baby". I shouted back, asking "Where was she sitting on the coach?" He looked at the woman and asked her the same question. She didn't seem to understand what he was saying, and what she responded, it was in a language I didn't understand. I think it was Polish. At that point I had an incredibly difficult decision to make. I knew I had to leave the man, to help find the missing baby. The guilt flooded over me, but I rationalised that I had at least stemmed his bleeding and bought him some time.

I ran toward the coach as fast as I could and took a final glance over my shoulder to see the paramedic I had just left bend down next to my casualty. I knew he was now getting some help, so I focussed on my next objective to find the baby. Having got to the coach, I could now fully appreciate the carnage. People where everywhere, ambulance staff frantically running here and there, desperately trying to help as many people as they could. Other firefighters were unloading all the equipment that would be needed to start cutting out people who were trapped, freeing them from the wreckage. The screams were sounding louder as I was moving closer. The closer I got to the coach the worse the people around me looked.

I remember seeing an elderly woman who had an arm torn from her body lying motionless in the road, a paramedic was desperately trying to apply a torniquet. There were children of all ages, some screaming and crying, others quiet and looking lost and scared. The scene felt completely over whelming, but I had to keep my focus. The only thing that was running though my mind was that I had to find the baby. I had no idea where the woman had been sat, what level of the bus she had been on or where to even start looking. I knew I had to act, knowing I was the only person with this critical piece of information and somehow, I had to get the baby back to the grief-stricken mother. By chance, I saw my officer in charge and quickly updated him with the information I was privy to. He ordered me to enter the coach to try to locate the missing baby.

The coach had come to rest on its side. I remember as I approached the roof, that there was a clear plastic hatch that the other firefighters had now cut through making an opening through which to gain access. It was very dark, I could once again hear screaming around me but this time I seemed to channel it out, it became a distant noise in the background. I could smell and taste a metallic type of aroma now inside, I recall shining my torch through the hatch and seeing people everywhere. It was very disorientating. As I passed through the hatch, I was climbing onto seats that were now on their side (I later found out the coach had 69 people on board). I climbed down and shone my torch into the darkness looking for any signs of the missing baby. I saw the tops of heads and people on top of each other or pinned by the weight of luggage, personal belongings like coats and bags. A woman was looking at me, stretching out her arms in a desperate bid to be pulled free. I bent down and pulled her towards me. I was only a few metres from the roof hatch entrance, so

I quickly passed her out towards the other waiting firefighters and medics.

Another two firefighters had entered the coach too and were helping to try and get out the people who weren't physically trapped. The other crews outside were instigating a plan to remove parts of the roof to gain better access to those who were physically trapped. I searched the top level of the bus, but I didn't locate the baby there. I remember thinking "please don't let me have missed them". I knew I had to keep moving and descend and check the ground floor. More confusion and more screaming met me as I made my way forward.

Finally, in the darkness I located the stairs. I tried to scramble down them sideways, which was a very bizarre and disorientating experience. Picture your staircase at home (unless you live in a bungalow), now imagine them laying flat on their side, and trying to walk down them. I got to the bottom of the narrow staircase and the scene was almost identical to the one I had just left on the first floor. I once again shone my torch around, but I could not see a baby, I held my breath and tried to see if I could make out the noise of a baby crying. I couldn't make anything out over the screams and cries of the other passengers. Suddenly, a noise came in over my hand-held radio, “we have located a baby”. I remember thinking “Is it alive?” “Is it the baby I was looking for or another baby?” How would they know? How would anyone know how many babies were on board? Should I stop searching or carry on?

Another radio message came in telling me to stay in the coach and keep helping anyone who wasn’t physically trapped and could walk with my assistance. This plan allowed us to clear as many people from the wreckage as we could, allowing us to locate the more seriously trapped and get them out using hydraulic and heavy lifting rescue equipment. Alongside the other firefighters, we got everyone out who wasn’t physically trapped. We knew a comprehensive plan was now in place to help the others and I was told to exit (the coach) and assist the ambulance crews with casualty care.

Once outside again the scene appeared even more chaotic, a lot of the injured that had been in the coach were now laying in the road, all needing help. I had never seen so many Ambulances, Police cars and Fire engines. There must have been at least 20 Ambulances, but clearly more were needed. The Police began to flag down and commandeer passing buses to ferry people to local A&E hospitals. It was a chaotic, frantic, desperate and traumatic scene and I have no doubt that it left its scar on everybody who attended that night, including myself.

I am pleased to be able to say the baby I was searching for was found alive and unhurt and was re-united with its mother. I don't know the fate of the first man I helped, he had been moved and taken to hospital by the time I was back outside. The worst thing for me about that job was the people we could not help. Four people lost limbs, two people died at the scene of their injuries, another died a few days later in hospital, and a large number suffered life changing injuries that will still be affecting them in their daily lives to this present day.

Nothing in my training had prepared me for the mental impact of this incident. I had not been given any tools to help me deal with it. The reason for sharing the details of this incident with you, is, so you understand what horrors we will almost certainly have to face whilst working within the emergency services. I want to share with you what support is in place to help deal with the after effects of such incidents. Back in 2007 at the time of this particular incident, there wasn't a great deal of support available. I remember seeing a few leaflets pinned to the fire station walls for charities or unions that offered help for stress, but I don't recall anyone using them. You would be asked by your officer in charge at the incident and once back to station 'if you felt ok', but that is where it usually stopped back then.

There was a bravado then of being 'superhuman' and 'strong', and not showing your emotions. It wasn't deemed 'macho' to admit to being affected by it. We were the ones that stayed strong for the public we served. We were often told by our peers we had to 'man up' and to 'get on with it', and so we did. I certainly didn't consider my mental wellbeing or fully understand how stress and trauma was really starting to affect me.

My crash

When I was 18, I was involved in a car crash. The year was 1999 and a friend of mine lost control of his car, as many of us did back when we thought we were all the next Niki Lauder's. We had been out at a local nightclub into the early hours. My friend who was driving wasn't drinking, we took it in turns back then to be the nominated driver, allowing the others to enjoy the night with a free lift home at the end of it.

We left the nightclub and the four of us piled into his car. I remember the roads were icy as we made our way home. We were only on the road a few minutes before we hit a patch of black ice. The car suddenly spun 360 degrees at speed, crashing backwards into a large tree on the edge of a golf course. I can remember the feeling as the car span out of control. There was no other traffic on the road and as the car began to spin everything seemed to slow down.

I remember gripping on to the handle above the window as we pirouetted down the icy tarmac. I was in the back, behind the passenger seat. A loud noise rang out as we smashed into the tree and came to rest. Then silence. I knew I was hurt. I was in shock. I sat still in the back whilst my senses absorbed the scene. I looked around me. My friend next to me in the back was trapped by his leg, it had become pinned between the driver's seat and the rear seats. The front passenger had been flung into the back seat with us, and the driver had taken some knocks in the front. Luckily, he managed to get out and dial 999. People from some nearby houses who had been awoken by the sound of the crash came out in their dressing gowns to try and help.

My memory is slightly blurry about the exact details of what happened next. I do, however, remember being pulled from the car and sat up against a nearby lamp post. I don't remember feeling any pain, but I was very cold, cold like I had never felt before. My whole body was shaking, which is the body's normal reaction to try and warm itself. I was in shock. I just wanted someone to tell me I was ok. A number of minutes later, I was loaded into an Ambulance and taken to hospital.

We were all discharged from the hospital the following morning with various injuries. I had some cuts to my head and shoulders from the glass and a very sore lower back. It hurt to stand up or to move around. Luckily none of us were seriously injured in that accident, but I had certainly been affected by the events.

A few days after the accident I remember running my fingers through my hair to feel the stitches in my scalp. When I pulled my hand away a big clump of hair came with it. I remember thinking wow, that must have been what they had cut away to stitch it up. I was worried, but almost out of reassurance or maybe out of panic I pulled on the hair near the front of my head away from the stiches. This also came straight out in my hands. I was literally pulling my hair out. I now felt genuinely panicked, I spoke to my mum who told me to phone the doctor. I booked an appointment and was seen the same day. My doctor explained that I was likely to be suffering from stress-induced hair loss. Something that is fairly common when someone experiences or is exposed to a traumatic event such as this one.

I had really been affected by this accident. I began to worry about getting back into my friends' cars, especially with the way some of them drove back then! When I did pluck up the courage, I was forever telling them to "slow down", "be careful", "you're going to kill us". Let's just say, I was told on a number of occasions by my mates, to 'shut up' and 'you really need to grow a pair'. My confidence had hit rock bottom and I was feeling anxious.

I'd been a happy go lucky 18-year-old, with no worries in the world, now I suddenly looked at life a lot differently. It took me a long time to reset my mind and regain the courage to just jump into a mate's car, or the car of a mate of a mate who I had never met without worrying about crashing again. Luckily for me, as time passed, the memories of the event lessened and faded and I would say I eventually returned to a state of normality. Well for the moment anyway. We will explore what this normality is and how our bodies reset a bit later on.

Losing a mate

In 2004, the year before I joined the fire and rescue service. I lost a very close friend of mine. He died in another car crash. This hit me particularly hard at the time. I was twenty-two and working as an electrician. It was on a Sunday morning that I had a phone call out the blue from another close mate. He said 'Gusty' was dead. He told me he had been killed in a crash on the dual carriageway, near where we lived, earlier that morning.

Gusty's nickname came from his surname Auguste. We had gone to secondary school together. He had taken me under his wing (as one of the much cooler kids). I didn't have much direction at school and certainly wasn't very academic, I stumbled my way through school not really knowing what I wanted to be when I left. My dad said I needed a trade behind me, so I left school with very few decent grades but with a drive to become a tradesman. Me and 'Gusty' would hang out together throughout our school years, and I got to know his family very well. We spent one whole summer holiday going out every day, doing what teenagers do, playing football, mucking around, getting into trouble and then going back to his house, watching films and falling asleep on his sofa. We'd do the same thing the next day, and so on. He also came on a few holidays with me and my family. He was very well liked, and had a huge group of friends from school, college, football and the area where he lived. He was a bit of a local legend, and I remember when he died the amount of people who turned up at his mum's house crying and grieving, this really showed me how many people's lives he had touched and was a part of.

I had experienced death before; all but one of my grandparents had died by this point. But this felt very different. It felt as though I had a part of me ripped away without warning. I had a good group of mates around me and we were all going through the same thing. So, we dealt with it the best way we knew how. By going to the pub and getting drunk. I drank to 'take away' or 'dull' the pain and used it as my coping mechanism.

There was a big pub culture in the early noughties, and we could pretty much hit a different one every night of the week. This took its toll on the electrical work I was doing at the time, I started turning up late, or worse, not at all. Drinking until the early hours and then trying to get up at 7am for work was not a good combination for me but I did manage to keep working, I just wasn't very productive and all the time

I was waiting for the end of the day so I could go to the pub and start all over again.

Around the time of Gusty's death, mental health and wellbeing wasn't on my radar, it wasn't something that I knew anything about, and I really just sailed through life without giving 'me' much thought. I had support around me by the way of a very caring family and great mates, but it didn't really help. I still 'felt like crap', and I really missed my mate.

The hardest moment was when I had to say goodbye. His family were quite religious and had arranged for an open casket ceremony prior to the funeral. It was in a local church and was just for close friends and family. 'Mr Popular' still had about fifty people turn up even to this! I remember his mum and all his family in tears, crying, screaming, singing. He was from a Caribbean background and deaths were to be celebrated in this culture. I deliberately tried to go into the Church on my own without anybody else. I wanted to say goodbye to my mate alone. People understood so I went in, it was very dark, there were a few dim candles scattered around the room. It smelt like a Church, that smell of incense mixed with damp. The coffin was open, and as I approached, I could see him lying there dressed in his bright blue football kit which his family had dressed him in. No 7 on the front - his number. He looked peaceful, but not as I remembered him. He looked really cold. I was holding back my tears as I chatted to him. I'm not a religious person myself, but I spoke to him softly as if he was listening back.

I remember thinking this was the last time I would see him again. He would no longer exist again on this planet. I remember thinking that it wasn't fair, I was angry and why this cruel blow had to hit our lives? I said my goodbyes and touched his cold hand before leaving him forever. This really affected me. For months after, his face was the last image I saw as I closed my eyes at night and the first image I saw when I woke up. His death was clearly impacting me, I didn't know if what I was feeling was 'normal' or not. I pretended to everybody around me that I was fine, I put on a brave face and 'bottled up' my sorrow and pain.

I deal with death and traumatic events completely differently now, knowing what I now know. My advice is never try to be someone you are not. Don't hide behind a false mask pretending you are ok in the hope that things will improve. This can be a vicious circle that will impact your mental health, causing suffering for you and others around you. I know that dealing with loss and grieving are very personal experiences and everybody will handle it differently. Whilst experiencing the grief and dark feelings that come with death.

Mourning for someone is a completely natural cycle of emotions and an unavoidable part of life. Another way of coping with these traumatic feelings could be sought by trying new experiences. The often deep-seated sense of loss can be dulled by exploring your creative side. Taking up painting or drawing, playing music, writing, or poetry are ways in which you can express your feelings and mood. These often compliment the way you are feeling and can serve as a healthy way of dealing with and processing grief. So, if you are dealing with grief, don't hit the pubs, instead maybe grab the drumsticks or paintbrushes, and use your creative side to support you in healing healthily and creatively.

Fact: *Did you know Sir Winston Churchill used to draw when he was suffering from depression?*

What will be the death of me?

I remember watching a documentary on TV about a group of misbehaving and troubled 16-year-olds who had been enrolled in an Army camp. This was with the hope that the experience would assist them towards becoming more mature and keep them on a pathway to success rather than failure. They were being put through their paces by a very menacing looking drill sergeant in his late 50's. He lined them all up on the squad line. But they were all smirking and laughing and not taking him seriously. He very calmly uttered six words that have stuck with me ever since.

'You are all going to die'. The misbehaving youths stopped in their tracks, now silent and were trying to work out this threat. Again, he shouted 'You are all going to die'. Once they realised that this wasn't ultimately an immediate threat to their existence, and he wasn't going to shoot twelve teenagers on national television. The penny dropped with them, as to what he was trying to get across. I also now understood the message he was conveying.

He wanted them to appreciate that we are not around forever and to serve as a reminder of how delicate life is and that it should be appreciated. Eighty plus years (if we're lucky), may seem a really long time to a teenager, it really isn't. The older I get the more I find myself repeating the drill sergeants' words of wisdom. We need to take time to stop, think, reflect, appreciate and enjoy our existence, it really should make you value and appreciate what you have got. In my opinion, this appreciation makes you a much better person.

I feel by valuing your existence, you are saying I value my life and I want to live it. You become kinder towards other humans, more forgiving and less inclined to hate. Pause for a minute, and ponder that in 125 years' time, no one alive on this planet today, now whilst you are reading this paragraph, will exist anymore. All gone, apart from a handful, most will be forgotten. Reflect on that. Really reflect on it, and only then will you realise or remember how important 'life' really is.

I understand why people are fearful of death; they don't want to die. The thought of how you may die can be overwhelming to some and that is why cognitively it is not always at the forefront of our minds.

An equally important issue to reflect on is, not to be afraid of death. Like I have mentioned, it will happen to every single one of us. Can you remember what it was like to be alive in 1782? Or 1882? Or pick any other uneventful year you like from before the day you were born.

Well of course not, don't be idiotic you must be thinking, I wasn't born yet to remember that date. As I have mentioned, I am not a religious individual, I am however spiritual, and firmly believe that life, however we got here, is very precious and should be respected.

The reason I asked you the question was to make you think. Why be scared of death? If we didn't fear anything before we were alive, why do we think we will fear anything after death. People who are religious may have an alternate view and I wholeheartedly respect that view. My point is not to fear death, but to celebrate life and respect everyone's views equally.

Part Two – Bang In Trouble

Pull over

If the engine management light comes on in your car, we know the potential consequences of ignoring it. A breakdown at best, at worst, a very costly catastrophic failure. We know that we should stop and as soon as possible ask a professional to take a look. The engine of your car is no different to our human mind. The thing is though, sometimes we don't recognise our 'warning light' or more often, and more dangerously, we simply consciously or unconsciously ignore it.

I remember that somewhere in my third year in the fire service, we were driving back from an incident we had attended. It wasn't anything serious, a fire in the open if my memory serves me. I was in the driving seat of the pump, my three other crew members were around me all talking casually. I suddenly became short of breath, I felt panicked, it was a very strange sensation. Nothing I had felt before. I was not in any danger and in a very normal no risk 'run of the mill' situation. I remember thinking to myself, 'something doesn't feel right'. My heart felt like it was racing in my chest and I was struggling to catch my breath.

It honestly felt as though I was having a heart attack. I looked into the big wing mirror and my face was as white as a sheet. We were only a mile or so from the fire station. I sat tight, trying to focus on driving without saying anything to my colleagues, in the hope I could get back to the fire station and no one would notice. I pulled into the station yard, parked up quickly, gave an excuse that I needed the toilet and jumped out of the pump.

I remember getting to the sink and looking at myself in the mirror; I was still short of breath and genuinely thought I might die. My heart was still pumping out my chest, my face still white as a sheet and I couldn't work out what was happening to me. I sat down on the toilet, closed the door and tried to talk sense to myself. I remember telling myself I couldn't be having a heart attack as I haven't got any chest pains. I reasoned to myself that I was a firefighter, who had undergone numerous routine medicals and fitness tests and kept myself fit and active.

A moment later the overwhelming feeling had eventually passed as quick as it had arrived, there was a knock on the door, "You alright in there mate? you need to put the pump away". I leapt up and got back to work. That episode scared me, and I thought about it for the rest of that day and all that night.

Some of you might relate to or recognise that experience. I didn't know it at the time, but I was having my first panic attack. I believe this was bought on by a combination of factors. We'd had a run of busy nights at our station and a lot of disturbed sleep. I was never good at sleeping during the day after coming off a night shift, but this was the time we were supposed to catch up on sleep and rest ahead of our next shift.

My diet at the time wasn't amazing. I was single and relied on the convenience of takeaways a lot of the time, as I was too tired or too lazy to cook, although I did exercise regularly. Our station had a very good gym with lots of equipment and so I did feel reasonably fit and healthy for a young guy. I was in a little debt at the time, nothing major, but enough so that I was living wage packet to wage packet, asking for subs from my mates or colleagues and I was worrying about it. The expensive takeaways probably didn't help matters! This combination of the stress of the job, poor diet, little sleep and the constant worry over money is, I think, what triggered this first attack.

It's happening again

Over the next few months, I was paranoid I might have another episode and the embarrassment I might feel if it happened on station, or worse at an incident. It did, a number of times! On one occasion I was at the scene of another RTC; a head on collision. Unfortunately, the driver had suffered horrific leg injuries and died before we arrived. We were tasked to remove the body from the wreckage. This is usually completed after the Police have investigated the cause of the collision and can often be delayed until a number of hours after the actual crash.

Alongside my other colleagues a plan was put in place to remove the side door, lift the dash board using a hydraulic ram and free the deceased man's trapped legs. We then covered him in a blanket and put him into a body bag to be taken by private Ambulance to the hospital mortuary. The tools were laid out and the officer in charge gave the orders; I was on the hydraulic spreaders ready to make entry when I felt that now increasingly familiar feeling. Shortness of breath, heart starting to race, feeling the blood drain from my face and panic rising. "Not now" I thought! My hands were shaking whilst I struggled to regain control of myself, the officer in charge noticed something was wrong "What's up" he asked? I didn't know what to say, I didn't want to lose my job because I couldn't do it anymore, or show weakness in front of my colleagues or feel that wasn't not good enough to be here. So, I shouted back "nothing boss", and I continued to try and regain my composure. This time I could feel it fading, and luckily, it did.

We got the man out of the car in the most dignified way we could, he looked peaceful. I went home that night still thinking about that job and asking myself why this feeling keeps happening to me. I was still visualising the face of the man we had just cut out and I remember so many thoughts going through my head whilst I lay in bed. How did it happen? Why did he have to die? What must his family be going though now? Question after question flowing through my mind with no available answers.

Then my attention focused on me. My mind still racing. What if I die in car crash? When will I die? What will death feel like? Will one of these panic attacks turn into a heart attack and I'll drop dead? Clearly these thoughts are not 'normal'; I didn't know it at the time, but I do now.

I now know exactly what is happening, why it's happening, and what I can do to stop it happening. Information I cannot wait to share with you, so you will be equipped to understand what can influence our amazing but often delicate minds. How you can take back control, and, realising that if it does happen to you, how you can just ride the wave as it will be over soon, and you will return to a state of calm.

I will talk about these coping mechanisms in a later chapter and why we should try and ensure we take a proactive approach to our personal welfare and mental wellbeing, rather than a reactive one.

Don't play Doctor

I think I must have experienced about half a dozen panic attacks over a six-month period early on in that early stage of my career. I remember thinking I needed to do something about it, as it was really beginning to affect my confidence.

I, of course looked online, I did the thing you should never do! The internet can give you thousands of answers, a doctor will give you the informed one. Do not pretend to be a doctor and start researching your own symptoms. Get professional help. I will detail what help is out there later on, but for now, Bang! the first result that the internet offered up, racing heart, shortness of breath…. you're having a heart attack. The same feeling of dread started to wash over me again, starting at the base of my toes, rising up my legs, the feeling of my blood draining. "C'mon, it can't be that", I reminded myself, "I've experienced this a number of times and I'm still alive!", so I ruled that out (for now) from my own diagnosis process.

My frantic searching from webpage to webpage eventually led me to 'panic attacks' and onto something that I had never heard of before called 'health anxiety'. What I basically believed then; to be known as a hypochondriac! My mum is the world's worse for this! I once told her

I had back pain from lifting weights and she insisted I needed to go to the doctor as it was probably some form of spinal cancer. She used to tell me that my father's back problems were the first sign he had blocked arteries and that my fate is sure to be the same. She is a big worrier, but I know she has my best interests at heart. That said, I would deliberately not tell her if I was ill, just in case she would start to trawl the internet for the information on the weird and wonderful tropical virus's I might have developed from that runny nose. The more I actually read about 'health anxiety' though the more I related to what it was saying. On this occasion I got lucky with my research, but I wished I had just gone and spoken to my doctor who would have saved me a lot of time and worry.

I would often find myself fearing the physical symptoms and sensations I felt in my body. Basically, we can get trapped in a vicious cycle of thinking that we are seriously ill or dying because of the symptoms we believe we have. Some people can spend years going from doctor to doctor insisting that something must be wrong, even though every test carried out by medical professionals proves otherwise. I am not saying that if you have symptoms, you should not get checked, a lump, a bump, a constant pain could spell trouble. But it is when these feelings are constant and end up consuming you, when the worry ruins your everyday life and basically spoils your existence; this is the time you need to get some help and take back control.

It is because of how these thoughts were affecting me I decided to keep a record and write down how I was feeling, I started a thoughts diary. Below is one week's entries so you can see how my mind was causing me unnecessary pain, suffering and distress:

Day One: I was on the treadmill in the gym this morning and my heart rate increased, this made me think about how there was a chance I could have a heart attack whilst running.

Day Two: I drove past the scene of a previous car crash I saw whilst off duty where the driver had been put into a coma. I thought about myself dying in a car crash and pictured myself in a coma.

Day Three: I had trouble getting to sleep tonight; I kept seeing the image of a man who had died at the scene of an accident.

Day Four: I took the dog for a walk this morning, but I was hypersensitive to my breathing rate; I thought I was having another panic attack or at worse a heart attack. I had to stop and kneel down whilst trying to control my breathing.

Day Five: I woke up in the middle of the night in a hot sweat, heart rate was racing, I started to take my pulse rate; my heart palpitations lasted around 5 minutes.

Day Six: We attended a fatal incident at work today, tonight I woke up and my heart rate was high, I could feel my pulse in my throat. I couldn't stop visualising the old man who had died.

Day Seven: Woke up this morning and checked my pulse and breathing; it seemed high so I thought I should go see the doctor today as I'm getting really worried I'm going to die of a heart attack soon.

Can you relate to any of these feelings or experiences? If so, then you are not alone.

Clearly these feelings are not normal, and for a short period in my life anxiety symptoms and a continued worry about my physical health had a huge impact on both my work and personal life. My thoughts were all consuming.

I did book that visit to my local doctor. They sat me down and asked what was wrong. I explained that I was obsessing about my heart rate and feel like something was wrong with me. He pushed his stethoscope against my chest. His other hand feeling for my pulse in my wrist. A few minutes passed, total silence whilst he listened to my heart. I remember thinking 'oh no something must be wrong, its been ages now and he's not said anything, it must be a heart problem'.

I could feel my heart rate increasing and my skin getting clammy as these thoughts consumed me. The silence broke, "There's nothing wrong with you, all perfectly normal" he said calmy and softly. "Are you sure?", I said. As soon as I said this, I immediately regretted it.

How dare I insult this man's expertise and expert medical knowledge. It can take up to 10 years to become a doctor in the UK and this man clearly had many a number of years' experience under his belt. Now here I was questioning that. I felt offended for him, like if someone questioned my rationale or decision-making process in my job. I apologised, but I knew the only reason I wanted to hear his answer was for further reassurance. His response, 'No need to apologise, you're as fit as a fiddle, now go and enjoy the rest of your day and try and be kind to yourself'. Those words stick in my head to this day.

It's true, we must be kind to ourselves and remind ourselves of this from time to time, I'm in a stressful career, I expect to be stressed sometimes. Ride the wave.

Every two years in the fire and rescue service we have to go for a routine medical. This involves, amongst other things a blood pressure and heart rate check. Even to this day I still get apprehensive when that cuff is placed on my arm by a stranger and inflated, the intense wait until it finally 'spits out' a blood pressure reading. I was told by a nurse at one of these medicals I was probably suffering from white coat syndrome, and I feel this was exacerbated by my health anxiety. It took me a number of years, a great deal of focus and energy as well as the advice like that contained within the pages of this book and others, until these intense feelings diminished. I must of died hundreds of times over and over again in my head, my mind was my worst enemy. However, I am still here, alive and healthy. You need to remind yourself it's not real and it's your mind playing tricks on you. My advice would be to think of a really strong role model and imagine if they were going through the same thing, how do you think your ideal role model would react in that moment? Once you master this and you stop worrying about death, disease or dying, you become so distracted by the good, you don't have the opportunity or care to worry. I have no problem getting my heart rate checked now, nor do I stress unnecessarily about my own health. Suddenly, all the phantom pains I was experiencing in my heart and in my body disappeared.

If you can relate to these feelings, then I would suggest you read a very good book that will explain this type of anxiety in greater detail: '***Stop worrying about your health'*** You can find details in the 'where to look for some help and inspiration' section in Part Eight.

I firmly believe we should all try to enjoy every single second of life, it is something that can be taken away in a flash and without warning. I have seen this first-hand and my new appreciation of this has helped me to re-focus my outlook and energy on life and ensure my wellbeing is given the respect it deserves.

The average person is alive for a measly 650,000 hours, if you are lucky, you need to use every single one of them wisely. Don't ignore your 'warning light' and remind yourself that worrying just means you are suffering twice.

Part Three: The Figures Speak For Themselves

Am I normal?

Quote: *You can't heal in the same environment that made you sick.*

So, what does being 'normal' mean? We all talk about normal, normal behaviour, normal ways of dealing with things. I clearly had no real idea if the way I was feeling was 'normal'. I had no one to compare myself to. Me, my mates nor my colleagues ever discussed the way we were feeling. It wasn't the done thing. Instead, we buried our heads in the sand and carried on hoping anything that troubled us would all magically 'go away' by itself. Well, let me tell you, it doesn't. You have to talk to someone to ease the burden and rationalise your thoughts and feelings, tell someone how you are feeling. Whether this be a close friend, family member, colleague or doctor.

It took me time, advice from professionals and some basic life adjustments, to enable me to reach my place of mental wellbeing. And you can too.

Working in the emergency services today, luckily, welfare and mental health is given more attention than ever before. Sadly, for some, issues are not always recognised in time, but help is out there. We are still working hard to erode the bravado of days gone by through education and taking proactive steps with regard to employee welfare.

In 2017, the mental health charity MIND surveyed over 12,000 employees across public and private sectors and found there to be a higher prevalence of mental health problems within the public sector, as well as a lack of support available for when people do speak up. The survey found that public sector workers are a third more likely to say their mental health was poorer than their peers in the private sector. Almost half (48%), of public sector workers also said that they had experienced mental ill health issues at their current organisation and had taken time off because of it.

An earlier, 2016 online survey of 1,600 staff and volunteers from Police, Fire, Ambulance and search and rescue services showed that 92% of participants had experienced stress, low mood and poor mental health at some point whilst working in the emergency services. A staggering 62% said they had experienced a mental health problem such as depression, anxiety disorder, post traumatic stress disorder (PTSD), bipolar disorder or schizophrenia while working in their current or previous blue light role. A more recent 2019 study titled Mental Health in the Emergency Service highlighted even more frightening figures. 76% of ambulance service staff and volunteers who took part in this survey had a personal experience of mental health problems. Nearly half, (46%) said that someone would be treated differently (in a negative way) if they disclosed a mental health problem to their organisation.

There is clearly much more that needs to be done. More investment of both time and money into recognising mental health in the workplace and clear pathways to help, must be considered an ongoing priority for all organisations. They must ensure they are taking robust steps to prevent staff suffering mental health in the first place rather than taking a reactive approach often, once it is too late. Picking up the pieces should be the last resort, not the first. Whilst it is the responsibility of your organisation to provide this support, it is equally important that you, yourself, take matters into your own hands. Take some meaningful steps to start looking after yourself, rather than waiting for help once the damage is done. After all, human beings are amazing. You are amazing.

A bag of tricks

Quote: *"You start to die the moment you are born. The whole of life is cutting through the pack with death. So take it easy"* – ***Sir Ian Fleming***

As soon as we are born, we are dying. From every hidden micro-organism to the biggest blue whale, the fight against entropy is an ongoing battle. This is explained in the second law of thermal dynamics. The entire universe in which we exist, all 93 billion light years in diameter and 13.7 billion years old, is on a downward pathway to its demise. This hypothesis explores that in the ever-expanding universe all energy is evenly distributed and therefore if it continues to expand will eventually reach the point of thermodynamic free energy. The universes would be unable to sustain an expanding process that increases entropy and heat death would occur. Despite this though, life has an incredible ability to battle this unseen force and bounce back bigger, better and stronger.

In the book, **A Short History of *nearly* Everything** by the world-famous author **Bill Bryson** offers an amazing introduction to life, that resonates with me and I would like to share:

"To be here now, alive in the twenty-first century and smart enough to know it, you have to be the beneficiary of an extraordinary string of biological good fortune. Consider the fact that for 3.8 billion years, a period of time older than the earth's mountains and rivers and oceans, every one of your forebears on both sides has been attractive enough to find a mate, healthy enough to reproduce, and sufficiently blessed by fate and circumstances to live long enough to do so. Not one of your pertinent ancestors was squashed, devoured, drowned, starved, stuck fast, wounded or otherwise deflected from life's quest of delivering a tiny charge of genetic material to the right partner at the right moment to, eventually create, you".

Beautifully put Bill. How rare and beautiful it is even to exist. We are indeed both incredibly special and lucky to be on this planet at all. So let's ensure we enjoy every bloody minute of it!

We are a living, breathing, bag of complex chemicals all working in unison to keep us, us. The complicated computer that is our brain, is constantly perceiving what our senses are alerted to, as either being a threat or a non-threat. What we encounter day to day, triggers our complex bag of chemicals to shoot into action, without a second's notice, to keep us alive. This turns on our 'fight or flight' reaction.

Adrenaline is released into our body, heightening our senses to any perceived threat. We then have a choice. Face this threat, or the safer bet, leg it. I was always told by my dad that if your outnumbered or the odds are stacked against you, don't be afraid to run (at the end of the day, it's my body trying to keep me alive).

How we perceive threat is interesting. I'm sure you will agree that people who, by choice, decide to jump out of a plane feet first hoping that a thin sheet of fabric will deploy before they meet that field fast approaching, or climbing that skyscraper to the top without safety lines for a selfie; or swimming with great white sharks without a cage are all, a 'sandwich short of a picnic'.

They call themselves adrenaline junkies, individuals who have had their 'hazard warning' o-meter removed and who thrive on the feelings associated with intense risk. That is obviously the extreme end of the scale, but, for those like the most of us, who don't get thrills from near death experiences, our perception of hazard and risk depends very much on our perception of the danger that is presented. When we are faced with a feared situation and stay in that moment until we return to normality, our brains log it as a learning experience. We learn that we can be in that situation and survive. If we are continually exposed to similar experiences our brain starts to learn that the situation we once feared, can also be safe. This in turn dulls the threat response and it will not be met with such intensity next time.

You're bloody normal!

The physical and mental effects experienced by us when dealing with trauma or a traumatic experience is our 'normal' body's reaction to an 'abnormal' event. This could be dealing with an experience similar to that which I detailed in the 'Heart racing' chapter or something else entirely. In the emergency services we often think of 'trauma' as dealing with someone who has died. A fatality. This is not always the case; situations are wide ranging for all of us. Trauma can be our bodies perception to something that is affecting it. It could be the loss of a loved one or dealing with someone who has died at the scene of an incident. Equally, it could also be what many of us face during our normal lives. An argument at work or home; or that feeling you get inside you when you are arguing with your loved one and can't control your outbursts of emotion. It could be a road rage incident you were involved in on your way to work or dealing with the news a family pet has passed away. It could be that call from the doctor informing you that a family member has been taken ill or when you are being told your house is being repossessed due to late payments. All of these and many other events are all traumatic life experiences that our bodies will react to differently.

When we are exposed to a distressing or upsetting experience, something called cortisol is released into the blood stream. There is nothing we can do to stop this. Just like there is no control over when adrenaline is released and you get that intense feeling strike you. Like adrenaline, cortisol is a steroid hormone, it is produced naturally by the adrenal gland and is a primary stress hormone that curbs functions that would be nonessential or detrimental in a 'fight or flight' situation. Brilliant if we are under attack from a lion, bear or wild boar. Not so good if we are watching a TV programme in the comfort of our home, or while we are at work.

The amount of cortisol released into your blood will be determined by several factors.

- How full is your proverbial 'bucket'?
- How much can you take before you spill over?

- How much is going on in your life, such as how many fatalities or traumatic experiences have you had to deal with at work?

If you have a lot going on, and your bucket is full, then even the smallest trauma can hit you like a ton of bricks. Essentially you are consistently topping up the levels of cortisol and this can manifest into negative impacts to our bodies. It might shut down the digestive, reproductive or immune system. This is why when you are feeling stressed often you feel run down and become ill. It can also result in a number of unwanted side effects, like, anxiety, depression, digestive problems, headaches, heart disease, sleep problems, weight gain, memory loss and many others. In Information taken from: **Mayoclinic.org – Stress Management**.

Cortisol should naturally start to dissipate after any danger or perceived threat has passed. Your heat rate, blood pressure and other body systems should gradually return to a normal state. After a period of around 30-40 days the Cortisol should have completely left your system. This is why I tell people that if they have dealt with a traumatic experience and are feeling numb and distant that these are completely 'normal' feelings. They are the side effects of cortisol that we cannot control. If, however, you are continually bombarded with stressful and traumatic life events, like many who work in the emergency services are; the cortisol does not disappear. Your bucket is constantly spilling over and the levels don't drop. This can develop into chronic stress. If you do experience a nasty incident at work or in your home life, it is completely normal to think about it after the event. It is important to remember not to 'play doctor', if you are struggling, please talk to a professional.

Why do I keep seeing this?

I can still remember my first fatality as a probationary firefighter. It was actually my first ever fire call or 'shout' as its also known. A young man who was driving a small Astra van, attempted to make a U-turn on a fast B-road and it ultimately ended in him losing his life. I assisted in his extrication from the vehicle. I remember loading him into the air ambulance, he was still alive but fighting for his life. I later found out he succumbed to his injuries on the flight to hospital. That was in 2005. I can still remember his face, the car and the van that were involved, the time of day, the weather conditions, everything about that shout is forever etched into my memory. I now know these feelings are completely normal.

My mind and body (although we should not think of these as two separate things, something I will cover in more detail later on) has processed that event but cleverly stored it away into my long-term memory. This is a self-preservation method, so we are not continually reminded of horrible thoughts. Once something is stored away to long-term memory. It can then be used to our benefit, when we want to or need to. I'm in control of how I use that memory. For example, when I was recalling it for inclusion in this book.

Problems occur when we have little, or no control over our own traumatic memories. When they keep popping into our heads when we least expect them and for no good reason. Out for a nice meal, bang, you're thinking about the guy you cut free from that wreckage. Going for a nice walk in the sunshine, bang, your thinking about the resuscitation you had to do on that child. You get the idea.

Unwanted negative memories will have a real and detrimental impact on your outlook on life. You may well start to notice a different you. Mood swings, irritability, anger, violence, insomnia, nightmares, impulsive actions, refusal to talk about events and an inability to concentrate or make decisions. Taking your anger and frustration out on your loved ones but not knowing why. These are just the behavioural reactions.

Physical reactions can include, lack of concentration, hyperactivity, exhaustion or using drink or drugs to numb the pain. Any of these seeming familiar? You are not alone. These are all very common side effects of excess cortisol zipping round your blood stream. How can we manage this? What can we do about it? Well, luckily, 95% of people's cortisol levels would have dropped naturally over the 30-40 day period after the traumatic event and you will return to normality.

So yes, it is normal to think about how horrible that last job you went on the day of the event, or for it to keep you up that night, or a few days, or a week later. But, after about forty days if you are still thinking about it, if it's popping into your head when you don't want it to, or your mind is racing in bed, and it's having a negative influence on you, it's time to consider getting a little bit of help. If you are in that 5%, who need a little gentle nudge to reach your normal state of happiness, that's fine and completely normal. It is probably because you have so much going on, on a persistent basis that you've lost a little bit of your ability to manage things and need some direction to get a pathway back to 'normality'.

There are lots of ways you can achieve this, getting the help you need, and often it's easily accessible. Most organisations will have a self-referral method or welfare contact who will be able to signpost you. You can also speak to your own doctor. If you are worried about doing this, for fear of time wasting or not wanting to be judged, then again that is very common. But don't be. Trust me, any welfare help you may need won't be judged or come as a shock to the doctor, psychiatrist or counsellor. They are professionals whose job is it to listen. They have a wealth of knowledge and experience. Anything you tell them they would have heard many times before. Any symptoms you are experiencing they would have helped someone else before. Don't ever delay getting help. The sense of reassurance you will feel the first time you ask for help will be euphoric and serve as a huge relief. Don't put it off a second longer. In Part Eight is where you can find that very help.

Part Four: Emotions Fading Fast

Noticing change

Being in the emergency services, and feeling being 'part of something' is an amazing thing. Something I am truly proud of. However, it has definitely changed me, in a lot of ways; for the better. Unfortunately, for others, the changes are not always perceived as positive. I have routinely been told I am cold hearted, or that I don't seem to care about other people's lives or that I don't show compassion in my personal life.

As I have shared in previous chapters, I have lost loved ones and a very good friend. Most of these were before I joined the fire service. The deaths I have had to deal with since, have felt different. It feels like death has become a 'normal' part of my job and life; and this has come with some consequences.

When I first signed up for an exciting career in the fire and rescue service, I didn't really know what to expect. Of course, I had some idea, I did some research. I'd watched London's Burning, Backdraught, 999 Emergency! Well, that's what I thought I was signing up for. The Firefighters, Police Officers and Medics on the television seemed to 'get on with it'. I could do that. Who doesn't want to be the hero! I quickly realised though, that it wasn't like the television, or the movies would have you believe. Dealing with trauma is complicated and very real. When I joined, we didn't get any training on dealing with death or understanding about how trauma and mental health issues may affect us. We didn't have many wellbeing measures in place to support us. Luckily, now it is a hell of a lot better. Albeit, in my opinion we as a society, still have more to do. Especially in today's often chaotic and judgemental modern world.

Most organisations in the emergency services now have lots of support measures in place to help staff. They recognise the humanitarian need to look after people, and of course the business need to ensure staff are not off sick but are in work, doing their jobs.

In my current service we have Mental Health First Aiders. Other firefighters and staff members who wear a green ribbon and have been trained to listen, talk and signpost people to help where needed. We have a Welfare Officer and support team whose job it is to coordinate staff who have been affected by trauma and put in place measures to support them. There are staff help lines where guidance and trained councillors can be accessed 24/7 for those who need it.

We work alongside charities that will offer guided meditation sessions for staff. We really have moved on in terms of support. When I joined very little of this was in place. In fact, as explained earlier, asking for help when you were supposed to be the hero, was a no go. This attitude modelled me into a different person from who I was than when I joined.

Slowly and surely, the more death and trauma I encountered, and there were lots, the more my emotions dulled. I no longer expressed my emotions. I didn't really ever feel myself crying anymore. To put this in perspective, even as a teenager, I used to cry watching movies, whether it was Dumbo being bullied or when E.T slipped into a coma. My ability to relate and show empathy was gradually eroding. I didn't really notice. I really only began to realise when people close to me died and I was asked by friends and family why I wasn't upset. Inside of course I felt sad, but I had built up a defence barrier that meant my body played its poker face. I could be watching the television with my wife, a romantic movie or a real-life drama and she would be in floods of tears. And me, nothing. No reaction. Sure, inside I would feel the emotion attached to the feeling, but on the outside; nothing. The more I was reminded of this, the more I realised I had become desensitised. The dictionary definition is 'make less sensitive'. That is exactly what working in the fire service had done to me. Eroded my emotions and reactions over time.

I knew this wasn't healthy, and I knew it was a result of a repeated exposure to trauma. I needed to help myself claw back that emotional connection. Do something to make sure next time Dumbo made an appearance I would be bawling again. I didn't get any professional help with this though. Something I wish I had done at the time. I just made a promise to try to reconnect with my emotions.

Now I was aware of the problem, I didn't have to hide behind a fake exterior. It does not make you a brave person to bottle up or avoid your emotions. In fact, it can be very detrimental to your mental wellbeing. If you feel sorrow or joy, then don't be afraid to show it. Crying is an emotion that is embedded in our genetic make-up. So don't be afraid to show it.

Walking through water

"Mental health is a daily battle, but I win every day" **Mardy Bird** – *Top 10 world US tennis player.*

People who work within the emergency services and armed forces can see some truly frightening and terrible things, things that most people should never have to see.

I recently watched a YouTube video that shared a story from a Police Officer who was forced to take early retirement. He was from traffic policing and starred in the show Traffic Cops. I urge you to watch this video, it can be found in the 'where to find help and inspiration' section of this book.

The story from this Police Officer shows first-hand how front-line emergency services staff suffer from PTSD, and this particular case, sadly led to a personal break down and having to leave the force. Something that is becoming more and more common on the front line. His story is an honest and emotional heartfelt exposé of the suffering he had to endure. He described how the public perception is that the roads policing teams' sole job is to book speeding motorists, something that he explains is very far from the truth.

He talks about owning an 'invisible rucksack' filled with death, pain, anger and destruction that he is wearing all of the time, both in and out of work. When I first heard that term used it immediately rang true. He went on to reveal how he believes every serving officer carries this with them wherever they go. He explained that he had to retire due to the build-up of emotions linked to responding to multiple traumatic jobs over time. He described how he would try and hide the 'invisible rucksack' to disguise being someone he wasn't, and he goes on to explain how his life was a lie, portraying the image of a strong level-headed, calm, professional Police Officer. Whilst on the inside he was suffering significantly, on the brink of self-destruction.

If you are wearing your 'poker face' and pretending to be someone you are not, it will eventually become too much of a personal responsibility to bear and it will slip. Our bodies and minds are not designed to live a false life. We are born who we are, we evolve to be the person we are through personal experiences, parenting, coaches, mentors, friends or family. The list of how we grow to become us, is lengthy indeed.

We are clever but we cannot trick ourselves or others into believing we are mentally healthy if we are not. Being poorly isn't a choice;

what we choose to do about it is. We must reveal our true self and seek out the cure to the illness. The purpose of that Police officers' story is to share his experience with others, so they realise the feelings they are having are 'normal' and 'expected', and that they are not alone. Sadly, very far from being alone. He reinforced that people who are suffering, must seek the help they need. They must talk and tell someone. It is recognising that mental health issues are an illness, like any other illness and years of medical science have enabled health services to put in place cures. The help is there. Sadly, people are often too afraid to admit to the problem and seek out help. I thank him for being so open and honest and for sharing his story. It wasn't an easy thing, but it took him on a journey to recovery, improvement and development of his wellbeing. Don't let your rucksack become too heavy to pick up!

Compassion fatigue or Secondary Traumatic Stress is a condition of emotional and physical exhaustion. It can lead to a reduced ability to empathise or feel compassion for others. It is the direct result of working for organisations that deal with trauma. Across all of the emergency services and armed forces, whether you are a doctor, a police officer, a soldier, palliative care worker, a nurse, a paramedic or any of the many jobs across this sector, you are likely to have been exposed to a variety of disasters, illness, suffering traumas and death. On top of being desensitised, compassion fatigue can exhibit a number of other symptoms including lowered concentration, numbness, feelings of helplessness and a lack of self-satisfaction, it can even manifest into physical symptoms such as aches and pains.

In many ways our bodies are extremely robust, however, in others not so much. As I said earlier, we are a bag of complex chemicals and it doesn't take a lot to disturb that delicate balance. Like desensitisation, you can do something about it. You can take back control. You have the power to recognise and react. Take positive steps to recovery. Get help and listen to the advice I offer in the coming chapters.

Dr. Naomi Rachel Remen captures this perfectly "The expectation that we can be immersed in suffering and loss daily and not be touched by it is as unrealistic as expecting to be able to walk through water without getting wet". *Source:* **Kitchen Table Wisdom: Stories that heal' Penguin, New York 1996.** We all have a lot going on and we are battling to keep afloat. Life is full of problems. But if we understand that, and take measures to address them ourselves, life can become a lot, lot easier and calmer.

Personal Trauma

Our fears had been confirmed, the doctor leaned over and said, "I'm afraid the baby has no heart beat". Me and my wife had just gone for our first scan following years of trying for a baby and months of IVF. We had both been dealt the most awful and devastating blow, from the elation of the IVF working and being told we were pregnant, something I didn't think could and would, ever happen for us both. We had already gone through a failed round, and this was our second attempt. Travelling all the way to Kalamaria in Greece for the treatment and both sacrificing so much getting to the point of it being successful. My wife was a teacher and therefore getting time off work to undergo the treatment was tricky, luckily they supported the treatment and granted her the leave away from work, as did the fire service for me. Months of healthy eating plans and bespoke diets, acupuncture and staying away form alcohol, all preparing her body for the treatment. And it was all in vain. The whole thing really took its toll on our mental health and resilience as a couple. I was angry, frustrated and blaming the world for our loss. She was sad, anxious and in mental and physical pain from the surgery to remove the foetus. It was all becoming a little too much and we both started to deal in absolutes. Our heads kept telling us that this will never happen for us and we should stop trying for a family. We would get frustrated with each other and that would turn to blame. We both knew that if we were going to overcome this personal trauma and fight back against the world, we had to do it together as a team. The journey had already been filled with suffering and mental anguish so we knew how strong we would have to be to continue on this pathway. We had to stay calm and focussed and remember our own wellbeing advice. We took a proactive approach to our mental health and used some of the things I've mentioned throughout this book to compliment our capacity to heal and grow more durable. We adjusted our mind set to one of positivity and confidence. It was so difficult telling people about what we had endured, deliberately lying or avoiding what had happened to us. We both knew telling our close friends and family would be a huge gamble, we stayed realistic to the possibility of failure, but they all knew we were going through IVF and wanted to know if it had worked. Having to go from delivering the most fantastic news and the joy that surrounds it, to the opposite is a horrendous task. Even long after, people we had forgotten we had told would remind us by genuinely and unmaliciously asking how it was all going with the treatment. We both knew we had to take the 'wins', her being pregnant in the first place was another step closer and something we thought incredibly unlikely only months before. We are still on this journey together and as yet; have not had the outcome we desire. However, we have been able to see it as just that, a journey, that we will overcome, together, as one.

Chest pounding

I have stressed how important I believe it is to make time for our personal wellbeing and development. The hard part is finding the time. I completely understand how busy we all are, but now is the time to take control of the situation. Stop making excuses about other influences on your time. We all have the power and the brilliance to develop our wellbeing to a level that will bring inner peace.

In December 2017 I was having a very stressful time at work and it was having a detrimental impact on my home life. I was newly promoted and in the middle of moving to a new house. I was suffering the effects of stress, but I didn't tell anyone about it. I kept it hidden form my colleagues, managers, friends and loved ones. I had little time for myself, and I was juggling lots of conflicting priorities both in and out of work. I was bottling up my emotions again and eventually the inevitable happened. I started to suffer from my ongoing health anxiety again. I would go to bed each night and lie awake worrying about all sorts of things. My head was a mess. But on the outside you would never have known. I kept my guard up and played my 'poker face'.

I now recognise that was completely the wrong thing to do. I had so much support around me but selfishly I choose not to accept it. I remember waking up in the middle of the night with my heart pounding in my chest, heart palpitations that lasted a few minutes at a time. It really panicked me. I could feel the stress pouring out of my core and filling my entire body with its negativity.

If you have ever experienced heart palpitations you'll know it can be scary. You feel as though your heart is pumping like you are running a marathon, but you are not, you are normally at rest. Heart palpitations are usually triggered by emotions or psychological issues, such as excitement, nervousness or stress and anxiety. In severe cases these can manifest into feeling nauseous and your limbs trembling. Your heartbeats suddenly become more noticeable, and you might feel them in your throat or neck. This will more than likely feel alarming, but in most cases, they are completely harmless and are not a sign of anything more serious. You may also feel an extra or missed beat, these are known as ectopic beats and are also nothing to worry about. It can be a combination of external stress and lifestyle impacts that can also trigger them. Not getting enough sleep, drinks containing caffeine, alcohol, drugs, smoking or rich and spicy foods.

The best thing you can do if you have experienced palpitations is to make some basic lifestyle adjustments and make the time for your wellbeing development. In most cases you do not need to see your doctor if the palpitations pass quickly and only happen occasionally. However, if you have a history of heart problems, they last a long time, or continue happening you should get them checked out by a doctor. If for nothing else, for your peace of mind and being able to return to calmness.

Making a promise

In late 2017 I was lying awake in bed trying to sleep when I finally made a promise to myself. I decided that I would make the time to help myself. That is when I started my wellbeing diary and thought about what proactive steps I could take to help make me more balanced and find my inner peace. I said to myself I would dedicate thirty minutes each evening to my own wellbeing. I would make the time. I promised myself I would. Why thirty minutes? Well, it seemed like an amount of time that I could commit to and maintain. I will talk about time management in a later chapter.

I looked at ways that I could find the time. What adjustments could I make to let me have thirty minutes of time dedicated to me and only me. What sacrifices would I have to make? Once I started looking at what my distractions were, I could work out which ones I could afford to ditch or scale back. It was a carefully considered balance of compromise. I wrote out all my conflicting distractions on one piece of paper, TV, work emails, personal emails, social media, house chores, looking at news, etc and how much time I thought I spent on each in a twenty-four-hour period.

On another piece of paper, I wrote down the things I wanted to replace them with. Guided meditation, reading books on wellbeing, listing to wellbeing podcasts, breathing exercises, etc. and I wrote down my mantra. My overall goal was to; keep a healthy work life balance, find my inner peace and take proactive steps to increase my wellbeing development.

I would encourage you to do this exercise. Find the time, make some sacrifices and get writing your list. On the first night I decided I was going to try a guided meditation which I'd found on an app on my phone. These can be searched for easily in your app store if you own a smart phone. If not, look online and there are lots of other options. I also mention some in the ‘where to look for help and inspiration’ section of this book. I explained to my wife that I needed thirty minutes each day on my own without any distractions. I explained my rationale and why it was important to me, she completely understood why I needed this, and she supported me. I think it is important that family members support each other when it comes to mental wellbeing.

I went to the bedroom, laid on the bed, put on my headphones and listened to the guided meditation. It takes a while and a bit of practice to completely let go and focus on you and only you. This is the premise of guided mediation; you try to block out all external distractions and concentrate on your own body and mind. After a week of doing this, thirty minutes each evening I already felt a million times better. I could feel the stress in my body subsiding. Like a drug I was getting a new high. High on feeling good. A high on life. Then I was chasing this newfound high.

What other adjustments could I make to benefit my wellbeing development? It was like a snowball effect, the more I looked at ways of self-improvement the better I felt on the inside. I looked at complimenting the guided mediation with some wellbeing self-help books. Then I started to read lots of different books all related to this subject. I also promised myself that in addition to the meditation I would read a snippet of one of the books each night before bed. Before I knew it, I had read eight books in a six-month period. Now I was really starting to feel the benefits. Each book offered a different perspective or opinion on how we can achieve wellbeing growth or spiritual development. I took a little bit away from each book and reminded myself of the key points daily. I wrote down the bits of each book which had the most meaningful impact on my wellbeing in my diary. I then used these to refer to when I needed a wellbeing boost.

Electronic heroin

Social media is a powerful tool. Something, that if used carefully and constructively can really compliment our lives. It connects us with family, friends and work colleagues, it can help us find a job or secure funding for charitable events as well as much, much more. The benefits are clear. However, another massive impact on our mental wellbeing is the overwhelming impact that some forms of information we take in has on us. We are constantly receiving information in one form or another. Some of it extremely useful and beneficial to us, some, utterly destructive. We get constant notifications and updates on our phones, smart watches, work and personal emails, through our electrical devices, the list goes on and on. Some of these notifications can bring us joy, it could be as simple as the sports team you follow winning a game or a post of your friend out celebrating.

Today we are so connected to the world 24/7 that filtering information is becoming a challenging test of our ability to switch off. We are at work all day dealing with issues and problems, often in stressful environments, only to come home and scroll through our various social media pages to extract from the dross, the information we consider important or relevant. We aimlessly scroll though looking at pictures and opinions from people we often don't know, getting drawn into often pointless and, endless debates on subjects we often don't care about. Opinions are like arseholes, everybody has one!

My own phone was set to inform me of news updates, so throughout the day and at home I would hear a noise alerting me, mainly to some disaster somewhere on the planet or an equally depressing news story. We are bombarded with information and unless its managed correctly it will cause us unwanted stress and anxiety.

A huge step I took was to completely come off social media. On a modern phone it will tell you how much screen time you're using on each app. It came as a complete shock to see just how often I used to visit Facebook, Twitter, Instagram, BBC News and other networking sites in a twenty-four-hour period. Most of you will be thinking there is no way I can possibly come off social media. Well at the time I thought the same. What about all the friends I wouldn't be able to connect with anymore, I would be sure to miss out on friend's birthdays and social events by missing important invites. I wouldn't be able to see what all of my friends and family are up to on a daily basis. I wouldn't be able to see their holiday pictures. It would be a complete disaster if I couldn't see what each of them had for dinner, or what opinion they held on any fairly typical political matter. Can you see where I'm going with this?

Social media plays a significant and important role in keeping people and businesses connected across the globe. Like it or not that is the stone-cold truth of the matter. Social media is a big part of life and is here to stay, it will continue to develop and move with the times. I remember in the early noughties when Myspace had millions of members across the entire planet, today, many people will never even heard of it. Trends come and go and the pace of change is quicker than most people can keep up with.

In early 2018 I finally took the plunge. My finger hovered over the 'delete' button on my Facebook account. Are you sure you want to delete your account another pop-up text screamed at me? You do realise you will lose all of your data, including photographs and memories. I pondered, but quickly reminded myself why I was doing this. I pressed it, it then took me to a screen saying don't worry we will keep all your data for 28 days in case you change your mind.

My wellbeing development journey had made my mind up. I didn't need convincing because my body told me it was the right decision. I was feeling great. So I deleted every single one of my social media accounts that week. I freed up so much time that could now be dedicated to my personal wellbeing development.

At the time of writing this book I have now been off social media for nearly four years, and I have not missed it one bit. I no longer feel any desire to worry about the detail of other people's lives. That may sound arrogant or rude, but it is not. If you genuinely want to engage with someone that means something to you then you can pick up the phone and call them or arrange to meet them. Don't think that 'liking' the photograph of them building a snowman, or a photograph of their cat, or what they had for breakfast, brunch, lunch, dinner etc etc is enough. These things don't really matter.

Trust me when I say that, for the majority of people their social media accounts are a way to mask inner anxiety. Most will post how perfect their lives are and how happy they are, when really, they are most unhappy. Most will post up a picture of their brand new expensive car but leave out the crippling finance they needed to commit to in order to have it. Most people leave out the misery and the dullness of what life actually sometimes throws at us hiding behind a fake digital mask of happiness.

People, especially those who are younger and susceptible to external influence who follow celebrities and social media stars can be made to feel incredibly unhappy, when they cannot live the life of their chosen idol. They may feel betrayed by life if they can't go on the expensive holidays or have the nice clothes that everybody else seems to have online. Social media rarely shows us the whole true story. We should all take a step back into reality and ask ourselves why we use social media? I am not asking you to follow what I did, you may use social media to support your business. My instruction is not to bury your head in the sand. However, the benefits of scaling back are clear, and your wellbeing journey would be greatly enhanced for doing so. Maybe start by taking a personal social media break. Try one day without any personal social media, then a week, then a month. For some that might be extremely difficult but imagine the time it will create to assist in your wellbeing. The benefits it has brought me are truly amazing and I thank myself for taking the risk. It has massively paid off. I urge you to try and limit your exposure and reduce this 'electronic heroin'.

The sad reality of the matter is that one day you might look up from your phone and realise the people you really care about won't be there anymore.

Part Five: Taking Back Control

Emergency landing

I liken the daily problems we all face to the holding pattern of aircraft circling above an airport waiting to land. Which problem are we going to let land first? Our minds are the air traffic control tower, processing each problem and considering its priority. Is that problem in our control; or does the problem need to push all the other problems aside and make an emergency landing, often without notice.

In the fire and rescue service I deal with problems every single day. Problem management and solving issues is what I would call my bread and butter. Something I consider myself to be rather good at. This experience has come from my time in the service and having been exposed to a large number of operational incidents. I deal with people on a daily basis and managing large groups of people can sometimes cause me problems that I have to deal with. Some are time critical, and a decision needs to be made immediately; others are not, and I can take time to think about and consider a range of potential outcomes to the issue.

In this modern world we are constantly bombarded with problems on a daily basis, some examples I have given in previous chapters. The hardest thing is not taking these problems home with us and them becoming the problems of our loved ones too. A significant amount of us work in stressful environments and more often than not, the problems and emotions associated with that work spill over into our personal lives. How often do you come home after a long day at work, or a difficult night shift and find yourself getting frustrated with loved ones at home? They can sometimes be seen as the enemy. The stress we have been feeling all day suddenly gets released to the very people we are trying to protect from it. We are tired, irritable, worried, we could also be feeling the effects of cortisol.

As mentioned earlier, you will now know how that little annoying hormone sinks its teeth into us when we least expect it. We finish work and arrive home, we now face yet more 'problems'. It could be something as trivial as making dinner or putting away the kid's toys. How often have you found yourself snapping at your loved ones or kids because they couldn't possibly understand how stressful your day was. And in your head, you want to shield them from your problems, so you end up not telling them. Instead, all you think about is how stressful your day was and if they really knew that there's no way they would be nagging at me to hoover up or drop the kids off at youth club. We should think of our home as a place of comfort and not challenge.

I have experienced this first-hand and it does not help our wellbeing development. We need to talk to our loved ones, let them know exactly how we are feeling. If we have had a stressful day at work, then tell them. I appreciate that some experiences and circumstances you may not want to or can't share. We don't have to go into gory detail. But it is important to talk about it. Don't keep things bottled up. Your loved ones will understand if you are stressed, you just need to let them know. If you don't tell them, they can't read your mind. It could be something as simple as having a code word for a bad day that each family member recognises as a trigger to show empathy and support.

Distractions

Let us say for a minute you are a working parent, if you are not don't worry, I just want you to imagine. You are consistently trying to strike a balance between how much time you dedicate to work and your loved ones. How often have you found yourself saying to your children “I’m so sorry, I’ve just not got the time, I’m so busy with work” or “I promise we will do that another time”.

Here is a typical day for you to think about.

Getting up in the morning, maybe a little late as you didn’t sleep particularly well, rushing around the house trying to get the children ready for school. Skipping breakfast as it got too late to make it, battling the school traffic to get there on time. Then the rat run through even more traffic until you reach your place of work. Then spending eight hours, often in a challenging and demanding role. Throw in the mix of being exposed to traumatic incidents during that time or maybe it’s just a difficult boss or whatever may cause you stress in your particular workplace. Then leaving to try and pick the children up from school on time. Getting home and working out how to get everybody fed and homework completed. You look at the clock, its already ten o’clock, where did that evening disappear too? You go to bed shattered. The alarm clock rings, and here we go again.

Sound familiar. Well maybe not for everyone but I would consider this a fairly typical example. Now throw in the mix relationship issues, being a single parent, personal health worries, debt, looking after ill or elderly relatives, supporting a friend who is going through a messy divorce, comforting your child who has just told you they have fallen out with their best friend at school. Now we are really ramping things up. Again, fairly typical for some. The list goes on, and people will have varying degrees of distractions all pulling them from pillar to post. They consume us, they take up all of our time, they constantly bombard us. Distractions are everywhere. We all need to find a sense of balance. A place where calmness can be achieved. Our bodies need it. We crave it as human beings. We have to be able to switch off and zone out.

In the modern society this is extremely difficult and only a few will truly master the balance, a real balance between work and life that achieves inner peace. This takes time, more time than you think you have, more time than you are willing to give, more hours than are in a day. Most people don't achieve this. They don't want to. They take the easy route and simply ignore it, being lazy or 'burying your head' are the easy options. This unfortunately comes at a considerable cost to their wellbeing. If you truly want to find inner peace and fight sedentary feelings, you have to give it the full attention and dedication it deserves. If you do, the rewards will be immense. Stop making excuses.

Striking the balance

Quote: *If you are in a bad mood, bad things will follow you. If you are in a good mood, you will find that great things happen* - ***Vex King, Good Vibes, Good Life, 2018.***

You are probably asking yourself well how I could possibly spare the time needed to achieve this, given that you have already given examples of where it would be impossible with everything I have going on?

If you find yourself asking this, you are already doubting it can be achieved. Well stop. Time can be found, and you can achieve the inner peace you crave. How nice would it be just to switch off and have no distractions? Time with you and only you. You will immediately feel better. A knock-on effect is that your relationship with yourself will improve, and in turn, your relationship with the world will follow. You will find calmness and loved ones will feel and see this calmness glow from within you. Your children, if you have them, will feel more loved, and you will feel more love for them.

I recently saw in the media an article that reinforces this theory. A single mother of a nine-year-old son, who worked as a nurse in an NHS department shared a story.

She said her son was feeling very low as he missed his friends from school, he had been schooling at home during the COVID 19 pandemic of 2020. She was working from home and very busy with work commitments, he complained to her that she never made enough time for him. Some parents would make the normal excuses that they are working hard but they will make sure they make it up to them. Some parents would continue to see their child dip deeper into unhappiness. Some would remind themselves that although it's unfair and far from ideal they can't give them the time they need as they have to keep working to keep a roof over their heads and food on the table.

This mother didn't make any excuses. Instead, she took a day off work, she stopped home schooling her son for one day. She told her son that this whole day is ours, what do you want to do? Anything you want. They watched movies, they ate ice cream together, they played board games, they dressed up in fancy dress, she read to him, he read to her. She said that the whole day he was happier than she had ever seen him and that night her son went to bed with the biggest smile on his face, as did she.

Some would say this was an irresponsible act. To make her son miss a day of essential schooling. Let's think of this another way. Her son was clearly upset, she wasn't giving him the time and attention he craved. He had no one else to communicate his problem too. He was angry and sad at always being told his mother hasn't got enough time for him. He was feeling anxious and suffering feelings of loneliness and isolation. What his mother did was both brave and innovative. She solved the problem, by dedicating her time. And I mean truly dedicating her time. No work calls, no checking social media, not quickly watching the last ten minutes of her TV programme. Phone switched off for the full day and the TV only switched on if her son wanted to. This proved to the child he was loved and valued.

This act would have had served as a massive boost to his confidence and security. He would never have felt better. His schoolwork would have improved, whereas if she didn't act, the distractions of him feeling unloved would have undoubtably caused performance issues in his educational development. She took a risk and it paid off. She felt more connected to her son than she ever did before. She made the time; time she didn't think she had. The result, improved happiness for her and her son. He finally felt valued. Valued enough that his mum took the whole day off to spend with him.

Mastering the sand

Quote: *You can't spell challenge without change.*

We sometimes need to use the time available to us to remind ourselves what truly matters to us. Why do I go to work? Why am I going for that promotion? Why did I want children?

When you are asking yourself these questions you are reflecting. You need to sense-check your life and your time. If work is consuming you so much that you do not have enough minutes in the day to spend with your loved ones, then maybe it's time for you to rethink your conflicting priorities. You have to feel grounded and valued as an individual and time management is key to achieving that fulfilment.

How often do you come home from work frustrated about your day and inadvertently and unintentionally take your frustration out on your loved ones? something I have already alluded to in previous chapters. This, again, is very common and can cause a number of issues in the home that have an effect on our mental wellbeing.

Every single one of us wants to be happy, joyful, embrace laughter and live full and meaningful lives. This, however, is rarely achievable all of the time, and it's more likely that we will find a balance somewhere in between total happiness and complete unhappiness. There are too many things that can influence our positivity and send us crashing back into a negative frame of mind. As mentioned earlier, it takes time and energy to truly give our wellbeing the attention it needs.

More and more people are turning to meditation as a way of finding inner peace, it is said to help improve focus and concentration, self-reflection, and lower levels of stress and anxiety. It does not work for everyone, and some people find it very difficult to completely shut out the world and only focus on themselves. I personally use regular meditation, and I would recommend that everyone that reads this book gives it a go. There are also other methods of meditation, included 'guided' that will talk you through the process step by step and is probably a good place to start if you find it hard to stay focused on your own. It may help you find your inner calm. In my 'Where to find help and inspiration' section in the back of this book, I will offer my suggestions and signpost to where to find some great places to start looking.

At work I routinely hear people say they can't find time to meditate, switch off or some other activity which allows their bodies to reset. We have so many conflicting appointments in our hectic lives, whether that be at work or in our private lives. People often find themselves making excuse after excuse as to why they couldn't find the time or why they couldn't go out for that run or go for a walk to clear their heads. Remember that, you, and only you can break the routine and find that time. Sometimes this can just be from an adjustment to your priorities. I cannot stress how important that is. If you want it, you'll find the time.

Part Six: Small Steps

Fighting the what ifs

I believe in something, I just haven't worked out what it is yet. As I have mentioned I am not a religious person, if someone asked me, I would consider myself someone who does not believe in God in the physical sense. However, I do believe in spiritual development and also that everything happens for a reason. Every knock, every set back, every unfortunate situation you can sometimes find yourself in. I firmly believe as human beings; we have to take the 'rough with the smooth'. We have to 'ride the wave' and all that it brings, until the calm resumes. We all want to be the best possible performers we can, as human beings we strive for excellence. We can be lazy, and we might try and take the easy route, but ultimately, we want to be classed as high performers usually through personal pride and wanting to maintain a positive reputation. However, we have to realise that we are going to make mistakes. We cannot possibly get it right all of the time and this often makes us ponder the what ifs and we spend time thinking about different outcomes.

PAST-----------NOW-----------FUTURE

Where on the timeline above do you think your mind spends most of its spare time? Do you think we spend our extremely valuable time living in the moment?

My career has largely been a very joyful and successful journey, however, like most, I have been impacted from challenging events both inside and outside of work. The higher I have climbed up the ranks within my own organisation the larger the workload and responsibility. This combination often comes with stress and worry about meeting timeframes and demand from senior commanders.

I have experienced setbacks in my career, I have been unsuccessful at promotional exams, I have not met deadlines because of conflicting workloads, I have made mistakes that have been frowned upon. I am highly self-critical and am constantly focusing on the negative aspects of my career pathway rather than, focusing on the positives, of which there are lots. This is through a passion for my chosen career and a commitment and drive to be the best I possibly can be. However, this comes at a cost, a lot of my time is spent dwelling on what I could have done better, or if I had only done something differently then the outcomes could have been different. I consistently give myself a preverbal beating, reliving scenarios over and over, causing myself misery and unhappiness. I rarely celebrate my successes and give myself a pat on the back for all my great work. Instead, my mind always reverts to negative reflection.

Reflection is critical to self-development and improvement, but not at the cost of mental wellbeing and health. I have learnt to strike a delicate balance between how long I reflect between the negative and positive outcomes. Reflecting on what has happened is often described by many as 'living in the past'. Trying to mentally correct what has happened in your mind, trying to justify and remedy the outcome in our heads as a way to try and change it. Almost creating a cognitive alternative reality to the truth. The reality is you can never change the past. You cannot in the present change or influence past events in any way. However hard your mind tries. This can consume us if we are not careful and we can become lost in a destructive mind set, only focusing on the 'what could have beens' and 'if onlys'.

The other end of the timeline is the future which can be equally distracting. We all know that planning and preparing are essential to life's successful pathway but too much focus on this can have negative connotations. For example, trying to influence on an upcoming exam, playing out each and every possible scenario in our minds, success, failure, what it would look like and how we would feel. Living in the future means we are essentially guessing what will happen to our lives. We can prepare for an exam, we can study, we can learn new skills, we can remain positive and focused. We can be hopeful for the best possible outcome but if we play out potential future scenarios over and over in our minds, this will distract us from the moment and cause unnecessary suffering, that will ultimately affect the time we should be spending in preparation for the exam in the first place.

We must try and remain focused in the present, of course from time to time we will sway back and forth from past, to present to future. But we must train our minds to stay grounded and draw ourselves back to the present moment. If we live outside of the present, we will miss what is happening now; right in front of us.

If that upcoming exam is looming, but we decide to go out for a nice country walk in the glorious sunshine, we may not be able to truly enjoy the experience because our mind is going through the destructive process of running though potential outcomes before we have even sat the exam. This will mentally remove us from the present, cause us suffering and will ruin our day out. Instead, we should have used our time to prepare for the exam, to ensure we are the best we can possibly be, reminding ourselves that we are ready and then if we decide to go for a walk to enjoy the present moment, living it and staying in it. It is a extremely challenging skill to master and takes a lot of time and energy but your life will change for the better. Meditation is an amazing tool to keep grounded and in the present. You are focusing your mind on you and your body and training your mind to focus away from the distractions of the past and the future.

You need to live in the present, enjoy it, for the next second it has gone forever. Don't let the distraction of what could have been, or what might be ruin what you are experiencing right now. Remaining in the present is both beautiful and captivating and it's this that keeps us grounded.

No one likes failing, or making a mistake, not at work nor in our personal lives. But we need to learn to make mistakes. It is the fundamental way we learn and develop as human beings. Embrace your mistakes, and if you are not making them, then often it is said that you are not working hard enough. You can start by taking small positive steps to return to the calm state before you made the mistake. Plan time to reflect, understanding reflection is a vital part of learning and underpinning future improvement. But reflection is also key to healing. Letting yourself off the hook. Plan for your mistake, remind yourself it was completely normal to make it, reflect on how you would approach it differently next time and then return to the present.

Carol S. Dweck, an American psychologist, captures this perfectly in her inspirational quote *"In a growth mindset, challenges are exciting rather than threatening. So rather than thinking, oh, I'm going to reveal my weakness, you say, wow, here's a chance to grow".*

Another detrimental human trait is to try and be liked by everybody that crosses your path. Again, incredibly unlikely. Your quest to impress and make everyone like you, will come at a cost to your own standards and your wellbeing. You cannot change people's opinions, after all, we are all extremely different and unique. If someone's opinion of you is not to their liking, then so what. Does it really matter? Moulding to other people's expectations or perceptions of you will only serve to diminish your sense of being and worth. Unfortunately, often the only person it impacts is you. You cannot influence everyone else. Instead, concentrate on yourself and control what you can, influence what you cannot control and adapt to what you cannot influence.

Battling stigmas

Many organisations worldwide are taking proactive measures in tackling the impact stress has on their staff. As I have already alluded to in previous chapters I feel more needs to be done. The emergency services have put in place some excellent control measures to help battle this often-unseen beast and are investing in proactive wellbeing and mental health services.

If someone is unfortunate enough to break their leg, we immediately know that that staff member will be off work for a long time. At least two to three months recovering from any surgery then often a lengthy rehabilitation period of physiotherapy and healing. We can both fully understand and comprehend that scenario. However, for mental health, when often the symptoms are far less obvious than a broken leg, the time off can be similar if not longer. The symptoms are usually masked by an individual's ability to disguise their internal suffering. I often overhear people saying things like 'wow that person is really milking their time off with this period of sickness' or 'how can you have so much time off for a mental health issue'. When someone breaks a bone, we send them flowers and cards. However, when someone is suffering from depression, there is sadly often silence from loved ones. We can't and shouldn't rush this healing process, nature sometimes takes a little while to do its thing.

Mental health cases are often complicated and not easy to understand. There is still so much we don't know about mental health and how it can affect us. We must remember it affects each of us very differently. We are all truly unique in how things can muddle our minds and impact our bodies. We need to continue to break down the stigma and educate as many people as possible of the signs and symptoms of mental health so we can all embrace the impacts and work together as a society.

Commonly, when people are lost to suicide, friends and family members are heard saying 'but they seemed so happy' or 'I was only with them yesterday and they were smiling, and you would never have known anything was wrong'. Unfortunately, suicide is becoming a lot more common, especially in younger people. Something I will talk about in more depth shortly. However, the point I'm making is people wear their 'poker face' on the outside and often work colleagues, family members and loved ones are duped into believing everything is ok. Often, that is the furthest from the truth. These people are sick and they are in desperate need of help. Help that is available and with time can cure the illness.

We must remind ourselves and others that mental health in whatever form that hits us, depression, pervasive development disorders, post-traumatic stress disorder (PTSD), bipolar disorder, anxiety disorder, panic disorder, phobias, eating disorders, schizophrenia the list goes on and on and are no different (in a hypothetical meaning) to a broken leg. The mind and body are broken, and measures need to be implemented for that mind and body to heal. That takes time. It often can take months or even years of therapy and professional help. It can be difficult to diagnose and often that contributes to the recovery time. Often, it can come and go, so it's not uncommon for there to be multiple periods of illness.

We all need to get smarter in how we educate people to reduce the stigmas in society surrounding mental health, we all need to take responsibility of showing compassion for this often-unseen illness. It's imperative that organisations continue to invest in education, so staff don't treat physical health and mental health as they are two separate entities, in terms of suffering and the impact they cause to the individual, they are not.

I was once challenged by a manager, condemning me for drawing a comparison between mental pain and physical pain, telling me 'they are absolutely nothing alike'. Its comments like these that compound the problem and often deter people from getting the help they need. Simply put we are whole; our minds and bodies are one.

Crisis point

I predominantly work in a male orientated environment in the fire and rescue service. The Home Office fire and rescue workforce statistics for England April 2019 to March 2020 reports that out of 32,171 firefighters across the United Kingdom only 7% (2461) are female. A figure fire and rescue services are not proud of and are working hard to address.

Having worked in this environment for a number of years I have come to a simple conclusion. *Most* men do not talk about their personal wellbeing, problems or emotions. Some do. Most, definitely do not. They often hide behind a facade of jokes, banter and false smiles. It is no surprise then, that when things take a dark turn and mental health problems surface, feelings and symptoms are bottled up and disguised.

It will be no surprise to learn then that the Office for National Statistics, Suicides in England and Wales: Registrations reports that in 2019, there were very sadly 5691 suicides recorded in England and Wales. Around 11 deaths for every 100,000 people. Around three-quarters of these were men (4303 deaths).

This is a consistent trend dating back to the mid 1990's. Males aged 45-49 had the highest age specific suicide rate (25.5 deaths per 100,000). For comparison, the female rate (5.3 deaths for every 100,000) is considerably lower. Suicide is also the leading cause of death amongst young people aged 20-34 years old.

Men don't like to talk about their worries and feelings. This is one reason why men are more likely to commit suicide than woman. Statistics from the same report state 72% of people who died by suicide over the last decade had not been in contact with their doctor or health professional.

MIND, the mental health charity has been running a 'Blue Light Programme' of mental health support for emergency services staff across England. In 2016 they published the results of an online survey of 200 firefighters. The results do not make good reading:

- 30% of firefighters had contemplated taking their own lives due to stress and poor mental health whilst working for the fire and rescue service
- 5% of firefighters had made an actual attempt to take their own life due to stress and poor mental health
- 61% of firefighters had experienced a mental health problem – such as depression, anxiety disorder, PTSD, bipolar disorder or schizophrenia

A report in 2015 was also commissioned by the Association of Ambulance Chief Executives due to concern against a perceived increase in suicide deaths amongst ambulance service staff in the United Kingdom. The aim was to determine whether these staff were at a higher risk of suicide than those who work in other professions. The results of the report found that:

- Between 2011 and 2015 there were 20 suicide deaths amongst paramedics in England
- The risk of suicide amongst male paramedics was 75% higher than the national average

- Over a two-year period 8 ambulance service trusts identified 15 staff suicides of which 11 were men and 4 women. The mean age of those dying by suicide was just 42 years old

Furthermore, figures from the Office of National Statistics highlight that between 2011 and 2019 more British Police officers took their own lives than had died in service.

169 serving officers took their own lives over this period, an average of around 21 deaths per year. By comparison during the same period there had only been 92 deaths on duty, an average of around 8 per year.

In 2019 the World Health Organisation (WHO) reported that globally 800,000 people die due to suicide every year. To put that figure into perspective, that is the population of Leeds. Imagine the equivalent of every man, woman and child from there not existing anymore; an alarmingly sad number. WHO declare suicide as a serious public health problem; however suicides can be preventable with timely, evidence based and often low-cost interventions. It recommends that every country has a comprehensive multisectoral suicide prevention strategy.

In 2012 HM Government published the 'Preventing Suicide in England' strategy. This details the governments tactical objectives of preventing and its commitment in the fight against suicide. It reported that, in England one person dies every two hours as a result of suicide. Suicide is a major issue for society and leading cause of years of life lost. They are preventable and there are many ways in which services, communities, individuals and society as whole can help support prevention.

The figures above clearly prove there is a high level of mental health need globally, in the UK and specifically within the emergency services.

Talk about it

Steps many emergency services organisations are taking to battle mental wellbeing are greatly improving. They have introduced a number of ways to educate staff on recognising the signs and symptoms that you may be affected by when experiencing a traumatic experience. If a firefighter has been exposed to a traumatic incident a specially trained officer will attend and carry out a diffusing session at the scene. This initial session is to make staff aware of the personal reactions that may be experienced over the next few days and weeks.

The reason for doing this it to ensure staff can recognise potential issues in themselves and others. They are then sign posted to support if they feel this is necessary. The officer will explain that people react to emotions differently and some of the reactions might not affect you at all. Some however, may experience these by varying degrees. They also highlight, once again, that traumatic stress is a normal reaction to an abnormal event and most often the associated feelings will dissipate within a month. A list of emotions that are commonly experienced are shared with the attending crews and these can include:

- Sadness, guilt, fear, shame or anger
- Anxiety and vulnerability
- Sleep disturbance – Insomnia and nightmares
- Isolation – 'no one understands'
- Lack of concentration
- Refusal to talk about the event to anyone

The officer will remind them not to be surprised if everyday things set you off thinking about the event and that you can re-experience the event through flashbacks. These can be triggered through sights, sounds, smells and taste.

Firefighters are reminded of the importance of sleep and the dangers of using drugs or alcohol as a coping mechanism. They are reminded that it is completely normal to have these reactions. There are encouraged to create a 'buddy system' where staff look out for changes in each other's behaviours. Colleagues will encourage them to seek help if they notice these changes. If the staff member refuses help, then the colleague is asked to share their concerns with a manager they trust or direct with the Human Resources department. They are reminded that if they ignore the issue, it may well get better, often it does, however it may also get worse.

We know a very small number of individuals do have persistent issues after dealing with traumatic incidents. They are given general advice on coping which I will share below:

- Try not to bottle things up – discuss any issues you have with someone that you trust
- Talk about the event with your family and friends – they will certainly want to listen
- Try not to isolate yourself – involve yourself in activities – live your life as fully and as normally as you can

- Try not to use alcohol as a support. A little alcohol may be useful to help you relax, however excessive amounts will have a negative effect, often disrupting your sleep patterns and will not help things improve

Staff are then reminded that if things don't improve naturally, then there is a range of support mechanisms in place if they need it. These include, but are not limited to:

- A trained trauma support team
- Mental Health First Aiders (a group of staff that have been trained to provide initial trauma and wellbeing support)
- Welfare Officer
- Employee Assistance Programme (this is an external provider where staff can access a range of confidential services 24/7 365 days a year)
- The Human Resources department
- Their own GP

In some cases a 'Trauma Support Debriefing Session' is carried out. This is where a trained trauma team will arrange to meet everybody who was exposed to the event and talk it through together as a group.

This process is proven to allow staff to talk openly with others who have experienced the same event, with a goal of trying to understand points of view of others they may not have been aware of and share reactions and coping mechanisms at an early stage.

During any traumatic incident the emergency services all have very different roles, responsibilities and organisational objectives. Fire service personal may not have a comprehensive understanding of the medical history of the casualty, whereas the Ambulance service will. We will also try to establish joint situational awareness but staff in more remote roles, like those working away from the main scene of operations, may not have the full picture as to why a situation turned out the way it did. We try to close this loop operationally by conducting a 'hot debrief' on scene. This is where outcomes are discussed by all organisations involved in the incident.

This is not always possible, because of the time critical nature of the work and it can be deliberately delayed. When this happens, certain staff will not be privy to the whole story and will rely on the information of others to 'close the loop' on their missing information. The purpose of the 'Trauma Support Debriefing Session' is to capture the gaps in the story. This process allows our minds to put the incident to long term memory and in most cases gives closure of the event. However, they are also reminded on rare occasions, issues can persist and often cannot be helped through the service. In these cases, the individual is reminded that additional more advanced support is available, and the service will work with them to identify the best pathway to recovery.

Helpful hints

These are some helpful hints which may assist you if you have been exposed to a traumatic event. Remember, as previously explained, a traumatic event does not have to mean someone has died. It can be caused by a number of things.

- Expect the incident to bother you and remind yourself that post incident reactions are completely normal
- Traumatic stress is a normal reaction to an abnormal incident or event and negative feelings will most often will dissipate naturally within 30-40 days
- Within the first 24 to 48 hours, exercise combined with relaxation will help combat any physical symptoms
- Watch what you put in your body, always try to maintain proper nutrition and be aware of the overuse of alcohol or

drugs to numb reaction (well-balanced and regular meals are important even when you do not feel like eating)

- Talk about your reactions to supportive networks like your colleagues, family and friends
- Continue a healthy work life balance, plan time for leisure and fun activities outside of work
- Get plenty of rest, however, expect that it is normal for your sleep to be disturbed for a few days
- Reoccurring thoughts, flashbacks, daydreams and nightmares are all normal. Try not to fight them, this is your body's reaction and coping mechanism – they will decrease over time and become less distressing
- Get additional help if you need it, talk to someone, there is a plethora of help out there if you need it

Part Seven: Reset

You're in command

Living the best life possible should be your new philosophy. Over two million years ago we were ape-man, we have evolved over this period of time into remarkable, wonderful and spectacular fleshy individuals with phenomenal resilience. We have advanced from an animal that had no cognitive reasoning to a race that can create music and the most incredible pieces of art, put people into space, climb mountains, design the pyramids and an infinite amount more. You are a part of something very special indeed.

It is time to take back control and bounce back to the person you want to be, happy, rested, confident, content and the very best version of yourself. There are no limits to our ability to have a full, meaningful and happy life. Welcome back to the best version of you.

You may have taken some hits; you may have received devastating impacts to your body and mind (as one). However, your journey will have made you stronger, and given you the knowledge and experience to be able to control your destiny. You can take back in control and ready to take on any challenge that is thrown your way and keep growing stronger and stronger one day at a time.

Every single one of us has mental health, something that is constantly with us. Just like we keep our body fit and healthy the same attention and commitment needs to be shown to our minds. We must ensure we take the pathways that continue our development and growth and not a route to destruction and death.

I have explained our continuing battle against entropy and how our own laziness can contribute to our poor mental wellbeing. Now that you have awareness of this, you can nurture the ability and strength to do something about it. That something, being, taking a proactive approach to your personal mental wellbeing, spiritual wellbeing and body and mind health. Develop your own personal mantra and use it whenever you need a reminder of your goals.

My advice would be to stay well away from gossip and negativity as much as you can. Of course, this is not always achievable, very few, unless you have decided to become a monk, can limit themselves from these daily influences. People who talk about others, spread rumours or deliberate hate are usually desperately unhappy themselves and use it as a coping mechanism. If we can limit our exposure to these impacts you will become happier and mentally healthier. If you hear someone spreading hate or circulating rumours, walk away. If this is on social media don't engage, turn off your device.

As mentioned in Part Five, you need to overcome laziness and master your sand. The ongoing commitment to finding time to develop your wellbeing. Start in small chunks and establish how you are going to use the time. What tools are you going to use to help you on your journey. Is it meditation? Reading self-help books? Wellbeing podcasts? Consider your options and ensure you aren't distracted from your goals.

Make sure your wellbeing diary is maintained and you write down everything that has inspired you. You can use this information to remind yourself of all the things that have encouraged and motivated you to grow stronger. You can use this newfound guidance to be the very best version of you there can be. Remember you are the world's greatest, there is only one of you who will ever exist. Treasure that experience and use it as a further reminder of how important life is, your life.

Keeping our bodies fit and healthy through regular exercise will have a positive impact on you. Remember not to distinguish your mind and body as two separate things. They are equal parts of you both connected working in unison to keep you developing. When your whole body feels happy, you feel happy.

So, what happens to our body during exercise? As our heart rate increases, blood flow to the brain increases. This causes an increase in both oxygen and nutrients. Proteins are also released; these keep the brain cells (neurons) healthy and promote the growth of brand-new neurons. They are the building blocks of our brains and as such are very important to overall mind health.

When exercising regularly, dopamine and endorphins are released in our brains, these are chemical reactions which make us feel happy. Not only do they make us feel much better but the brain is also getting rid of other chemicals which make us feel stressed, such as the dreaded cortisol. It is a well-known fact that people who maintain regular fitness are much more likely to feel happier and less stressed than those who don't. In addition to this, if you are having a bad time and are experiencing negativity, exercise will help regulate emotions such as feeling low, angry or upset.

Equally as important as regular exercise is undisturbed and restful sleep. Something we often take for granted. Another detrimental impact of social media is how often we find ourselves on it just before going to sleep. Ongoing research about the impact artificial light has on our bodies shows it has an effect on our circadian rhythms (your body clock) and in turn our metabolism. It suppresses our natural melatonin production; this is the hormone that helps induce sleep. You should look to impose an 'electronic shutdown' and not look at any electronic device for at least ninety minutes before sleeping. This will help you achieve a deeper and more relaxing sleep, and you will be more likely to wake up feeling both refreshed and happy.

Another addition to compliment your sleep could be trying out a pillow mist or a scented diffuser. There are several products on the market that are designed specifically to help you drift off to sleep more peacefully, reduce sleep anxiety and improve sleep quality. Give one a go if you are having trouble sleeping, you have nothing to lose, but everything to gain if it works for you.

My wife and I decided to take a well-earned relaxing break to the Cotswolds. I found a lovely quaint, contemporary hotel and booked two nights away. We were both going through a stressful time at work and in our personal lives, so we felt it was well deserved. I drove through the grounds and up the pebble driveway to the grade two listed building and was taken aback by its beauty and grandeur. We arrived in the reception area, checked in, and were taken up to our room. The moment I stepped inside the hotel room I felt immediately relaxed, I could feel the negativity leaving my body.

The room had a four-poster bed, free standing bathtub in the centre of the room and the décor was beautifully furnished. The most vivid memory I have from the whole experience is of laying on the bed, completely zoning out and listing to classical music coming from a radio on the bedside table. I had found my happy place. I could feel the stress leaving my body, pleasure and calm its replacement. We both agreed it was the most relaxed we had both felt in a very long time.

I wanted to try and replicate the experience at home. Now, every night after I have spent thirty minutes of dedicated wellbeing development, reading, meditating, breathing exercises or listing to podcasts. I turn on the radio I bought for our bedside table and put on Classic FM. This takes me back and reminds me of the relaxing state I was in in the hotel and lifts my mood. It also allows me to drift off to soothing, relaxing music. This is now my bedtime routine and I find my sleep to be peaceful, undisturbed, and complete.

If you were lucky enough to own one, you would not fill up your Ferrari sports car with diesel. The same consideration and choice should be given to your body. We must ensure we eat healthy foods and maintain a balanced diet. I am not going to tell you what you should and shouldn't eat. There is a mountain of information on nutritional advice if you wish to seek it out. Instead, all I would remind you is to evaluate what good food you eat against the bad stuff. If you eat a good diet, it will compliment all the other areas of your commitment to wellbeing that you have dedicated your precious time to and will make you feel even greater.

A good rule of thumb to stick too is the 80/20 compromise. Eat nutritious food 80% of the time, whilst the other 20% you can treat yourself. If you have eaten well all week and decide when the weekend arrives to treat yourself to a takeaway. Go for it. However, when you treat yourself, do not regret it. If you do, eating it will make you unhappy and will defy the point of eating it in the first place.

Is it healthy to dwell in the past? I have already mentioned the importance of reflection for developing growth and assisting in pathways to success. The habits of living in memories instead of staying grounded in the present can be detrimental. However, a healthy balance needs to be struck between past happy memories and those that are not complementing our personal development.

Nostalgia was considered a psychological disorder in the 17-century mainly due to the impact on a soldier's state of mind. Regarded as a condition of homesickness, an avoidance of the here and now and a longing for what has been lost, security, happiness and loved ones. In 1688 Johannes Hofer was a Swiss physician and he first coined the term. Home – *nostos* in Greek, and *algos*, meaning pain. According to Hofer, Swiss mercenaries serving abroad were particularly susceptible to bouts of nostalgia, especially when reminded of the sights, sounds and tastes of home. By the 18-Century nostalgia was no longer a provincial disease, over time it had become less of an acute homesickness for a specific place and more a sentimental longing for the past. *Reference*: David Anderson, Senior lecturer in American History. The soldiers who died of homesickness.

Using nostalgia to revisit happy memories of the past has helped my overall wellbeing and can be used as a tool to make life more meaningful. It can be a powerful escapism tool. A way of distraction and relief from realities. I'm very lucky to have fond memories of my childhood, I know some people are not always able to say that. Happy memories are important to our wellbeing, even if they are few and far between. Try and think back to your happiest childhood memory, what where you doing? Who were you with? Where were you?

Sensory triggers are also a great way of boosting your frame of mind, music is very powerful and playing songs from your adolescence or memorable happy moments can help release that 'feel good chemical' dopamine. Some of the other practical steps I take to heighten my nostalgic mood from time to time are by re-watching childhood TV programmes, adverts and films. I also recently purchased an original Gameboy, a retro handheld console, it felt fantastic to play some of the games from my childhood. Although the graphics are not quite up to today's standards (that's a bit of an understatement) it really did take me back to a happier place. Sharing these happy memories with loved ones can also make couples feel closer and more connected. All of these suggestions can complement your wellbeing development and assist in your pathway to happiness.

Final Words

Once again, thank you for taking your precious time to read this book. I hope you are now on a pathway to a calmer and more grounded you. As I have mentioned, life is very special indeed. Make sure you take a little time to reflect each day to remind yourself of that and use that reflection to empower your growth and wellbeing development. Life can sometimes throw a monumental amount of crap at you from time to time, but you have the power and the strength to anticipate this impact, use the guidance and tools I have mentioned to regain command. Strive for your own improvement and don't chase perfection. No one on this earth is perfect, you may believe everyone else has it better than you, but they do not. We are social creatures, and we want to 'fit in' and be liked, but my advice is stop trying to be someone you are not just to impress others around you. Keep your attention focused on your own wellbeing and socialise with people who compliment your pathway and not dismantle it.

Finally, we now know our life on this planet is extremely rare and we must use our time wisely. My advice would be to experience as much as you can and do the things that lift your mood. Be at one with nature, look up at the stars, watch the sunrise, read a great book, play with your pets, eat that big dessert, be silly, be compassionate, be caring, stop and help someone in need and be the best version of you, you can be. Have a think about what are your key elements to happiness? Now it's time to take your wellbeing to the next level and remember, be kind to yourself, always.

The Signs to look out for

Warning signs and red flags to look out for in your friends, family and colleagues:

- Talking about wanting to die
- Suggesting their life has no purpose or future
- Withdrawing or feeling isolated
- Talking about being a burden to others
- Experiencing extreme mood swings, irritability or anger
- Drug or alcohol misuse
- Feelings of hopelessness or disconnection
- Giving away possessions or writing a will
- Giving up previously loved activities or hobbies

This list is not exhaustive, be guided by you own instincts.

Part Eight: Where To Look For Help And Inspiration

Quote: *"it's ok to ask for some help"*

There are a wealth of places you can find self-help. If you take the time to look for it, you will find it. Listed below are some important contact numbers and useful suggestions of resources that have really helped compliment my wellbeing journey.

Speak to someone:

Tell one of your family, close friends or managers at work – It will be the hardest thing you do, but once you ask for help, I promise it will feel a huge relief. The hardest thing is to be honest to yourself and in turn honest to others. Don't try and cover it up. Speak to someone, they will listen.

Your Doctor – they can signpost you to the most appropriate support department.

Hospital – If you are having dark thoughts call 111 (NHS helpline) and ask for help, they might think you need immediate help and will either ask you to go to hospital or call you an ambulance. Remember if you feel out of control and it is that bad, help is available. Don't feel ashamed, you aren't the first person to go through this, it is much more common than you think. Go get that help and allow them to support you.

There are lots of voluntary organisations that can help people who are suffering with mental health issues, some of the ones I have found useful include:

MIND 0300 123 3393 www.mind.org

Samaritans 116 123 www.samaritians.org

CALM 0800 585858 www.thecalmzone.net

Papyrus 0800 068 4141 **www.papyrus-uk**

SHOUT text: 85258 www.giveusashout.org

The Firefighters Charity www.firefighterscharity.org.uk

NHS Urgent mental health support 24/7 –

nhs.uk/urgentmentalhealth

Books:

A few of the books that have really supported my pathway to calmness.

A Road Less Travelled – Scott Peck

Good Life Good Vibes – Vex King

Happy – Fearne Cotton

The Little Book of Ikigai – Ken Mogi

Stop worrying about your health - For people that have a unhealthy fear of dying (chapter three) George D. Zgourides

Why Has Nobody Told Me This Before? - Dr.Julie Smith

Podcasts and Downloads

Health Anxiety Show (The Anxiety Guy) Podcast

Headspace www.headspace.com

GABA – Guided meditation @gaba.life Podcast

Calm- Guided meditation www.calm.com

Happy Place – Ferne Cotton

Dad Still Standing Podcast

Inspiring watches:

The Job that BROKE ME retired Police officer (YouTube)

Acknowledgements

Sophie, my wife, my best friend, thank you, you gave me the support and encouragement to write this book. My family, friends and work colleagues who dedicated many hours and energy reading my many failed chapter attempts and providing me with invaluable feedback. Spiffing Covers for the amazing book cover design. And finally, I'd like to thank myself, which I don't do often enough, for believing in myself to make this a reality.

"None of us are getting out of here alive, so please stop treating yourself like an afterthought. Eat the delicious food. Walk in the sunshine. Jump in the ocean. Say the truth that you're carrying in your heart like hidden treasure. Be silly. Be kind. Be weird. There's no time for anything else" – **Sir Anthony Hopkins**

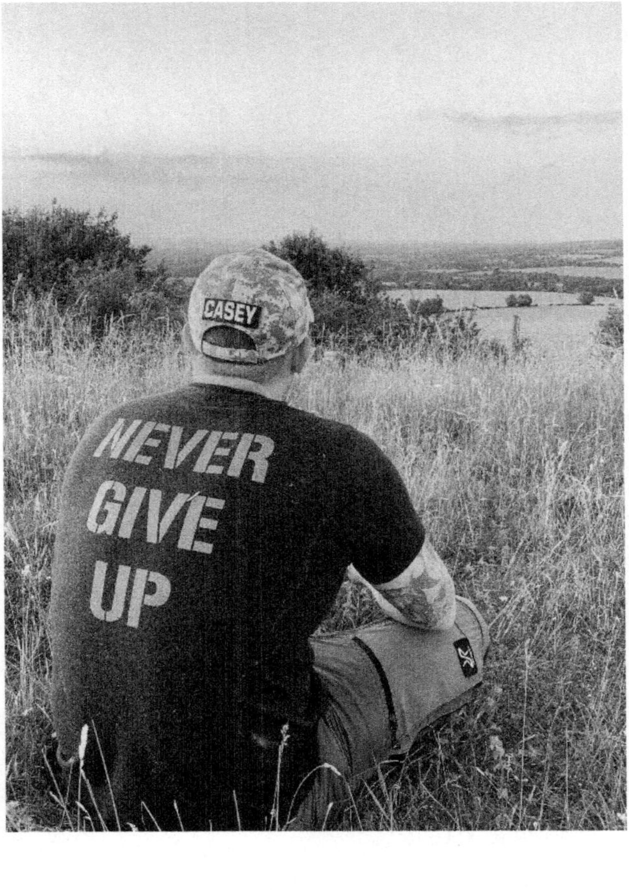
CASEY
NEVER
GIVE
UP

Printed in Great Britain
by Amazon

84067064R00071